Samuel Elisha Woody

The essentials of medical chemistry and urinalysis

Samuel Elisha Woody

The essentials of medical chemistry and urinalysis

ISBN/EAN: 9783742805751

Manufactured in Europe, USA, Canada, Australia, Japa

Cover: Foto ©Lupo / pixelio.de

Manufactured and distributed by brebook publishing software (www.brebook.com)

Samuel Elisha Woody

The essentials of medical chemistry and urinalysis

THE ESSENTIALS

OF

MEDICAL CHEMISTRY

AND

URINALYSIS.

BY

SAM E. WOODY, A. M., M. D.,

PROFESSOR OF CHEMISTRY AND PUBLIC HYGIENE, AND CLINICAL LECTURER ON DISEASES
OF CHILDREN, IN THE KENTUCKY SCHOOL OF MEDICINE.

THIRD EDITION,
REVISED, ENLARGED AND ILLUSTRATED.

PHILADELPHIA:
P. BLAKISTON, SON & CO.,
1012 WALNUT STREET.
1890.

Copyright, 1890, by P. Blakiston, Son & Co.

PRESS OF WM. F. FELL & CO.
1220 24 SANSOM STREET,
PHILADELPHIA.

PREFACE.

The THIRD EDITION treading so closely on the heels of its predecessors, assures the writer that his little book has found use in the hands of many medical students, and that his labor has lessened theirs.

As long as the effort is made to crowd the whole science of medicine into a five months' course, the hurried student must have such a book as this to present the *essential facts*, so that he need not wade through the more exhaustive text-books, or be compelled to take voluminous notes, which are unavoidably inaccurate and unsatisfactory. The selection of material and the plan of presentation is the outgrowth of the author's experience as a general practitioner and as a teacher of medical chemistry for the past twelve years.

The subjects treated are so numerous that the descriptions are necessarily brief, but the principles of the science and the application of the facts to medicine have been stated more fully.

1506 WEST WALNUT STREET,
    LOUISVILLE, KY.

CONTENTS.

	PAGE
INTRODUCTION,	9
Table of Elementary Bodies, with their Symbols and Atomic Weights,	12

PART I.—INORGANIC CHEMISTRY, ... 15

CLASSIFICATION OF THE ELEMENTS, ... 15

    I. Hydrogen and Oxygen Group, ... 16
        Hydrogen, 16. Oxygen, 17. Compounds of Hydrogen with Oxygen—Water, 20. Table of Valence, 27.

    II. The Chlorine Group, ... 28
        Fluorine, Chlorine, Bromine, Iodine, 28.

    III. The Sulphur Group, ... 34
        Sulphur, 35.

    IV. The Nitrogen Group, ... 40
        Nitrogen, 40. The Atmosphere, 41. Phosphorus, 46. Arsenic, 49. Antimony, 53. Bismuth, 55.

    V. The Carbon Group, ... 56
        Carbon, 56. Silicon, 61. Tin, 62. Lead, 63.

    VI. Metals of the Alkalies, ... 65
        Lithium, 65. Ammonium, 66. Sodium, 67. Potassium, 68. Cæsium and Rubidium, 71.

    VII. Metals of the Alkaline Earths, ... 71
        Magnesium, 71. Calcium, 73. Strontium, 75. Barium, 75.

    VIII. Metals of the Earths, ... 75
        Boron, 76. Aluminium, 76. Cerium, 77.

    IX. The Zinc Group, ... 77
        Zinc, 77. Cadmium, 79.

    X. The Iron Group, ... 79
        Chromium, 79. Manganese, 80. Iron, 81. Cobalt, 85. Nickel, 85.

CONTENTS.

	PAGE
XI. The Copper Group,	85
Copper, 85. Mercury, 87.	
XII. The Silver Group,	91
Silver, 91. Gold, 92. Platinum, 93.	
Table to Determine the Metallic Radical of a Salt,	94
Table to Determine the Acidulous Radical of a Salt,	95
Table—The Solubility or Insolubility of Salts in Water,	96

PART II.—ORGANIC CHEMISTRY, ... 97
  Hydrocarbons, ... 98
  Alcohols, ... 101
  Ethers, ... 105
  Aldehydes, ... 108
  Organic Acids, ... 109
  The Carbohydrates, ... 112
  Glucosides, ... 115
  Nitrogenous Bodies, ... 116
  Alkaloids, ... 118

PART III.—THE URINE, ... 121
  Physical Properties, ... 122
  Chemical Constituents, ... 126
  Tests for Albumin, etc., ... 133

THE ESSENTIALS OF
MEDICAL CHEMISTRY.

INTRODUCTION.

"Chemistry is that branch of science which treats of the composition of substances, their changes in composition and the laws governing such changes." (*Webster*.)

The distinctive characteristic of chemical action is change in *composition*.* A bar of iron is the same in composition, whether hot or cold, luminous or non-luminous, magnetized or unmagnetized. But when it undergoes chemical action a new substance is formed which, though it contains iron, is entirely different from it in composition and properties.†

Matter is that of which the sensible universe is composed. It is *indestructible*. Substances may undergo many changes, assume a great variety of forms, and even become invisible gases. Yet in none of these changes and combinations can a particle of matter be created or destroyed.‡ All matter has *weight*. By balances in the

---

* Experiment.—Heat pieces of platinum and magnesium wire. Note that while the platinum is unaltered the magnesium burns and is converted into a white powder of magnesium oxide.

† Experiment.—Weigh a small porcelain crucible containing powdered iron. Heat it, and it ignites; when combustion is complete, weigh again, and note the increase of weight and that a new substance is formed, which, though it contains iron, is not iron.

‡ Experiment.—Burn a piece of charcoal (carbon) in a jar of oxygen gas. (Fig. 1.) It disappears and, so far as we can judge by the senses of sight and touch, is lost, for it has combined with the oxygen to form an invisible gas. Add lime-water and shake. The gas combines with the lime and forms a white precipitate, which, if gathered and weighed, would exactly represent, besides the lime, the charcoal burned and the oxygen required to burn it.

open air we get the *apparent weight* of a body; but to obtain the *absolute weight* it must be weighed in a vacuum where there is no air to buoy it up. (For measures of weight, see table at back of book.) But of most importance to the student of chemistry is the *specific weight* or *specific gravity*, by which we mean the weight of a substance as compared to the weight of an equal volume of some other substance specified as a standard. The standard for solids and liquids is water; for gases, air or hydrogen.*

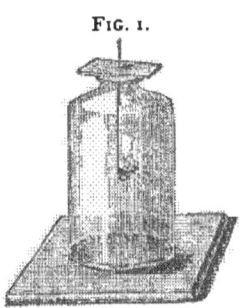

Fig. 1.

Matter exists in one of three states, solid, liquid, or gaseous. In the solid state the particles are held together

---

* The specific gravity of solids is determined on the principle of Archimedes: *A body immersed in a liquid displaces its own volume, and loses weight equal to the weight of the liquid displaced.* Therefore, the weight a body loses when weighed in water, is the weight of its own volume of water and the standard with which the weight of that body must be compared. For example, suppose

A piece of iron weighs	. . . .	150 grains.
Suspended in water it weighs	. . . .	130 grains.
Loss (or weight of its volume of water)	. . .	20 grains.
Specific gravity of the iron (150 ÷ 20)	. . .	7.5

In case the body is lighter than water, a sinker is attached and the same method pursued, except that the loss of weight of the sinker is also obtained separately and subtracted from the total loss to ascertain the loss of weight of the lighter body. A body soluble in water may be weighed in some liquid of known specific gravity in which it is insoluble; *e. g.*, suppose a lump of sugar weighs 100 grains, and in turpentine 45.62 grains. Loss = 100 − 45.62 = 54.38 grains. 100 ÷ 54.38 = 1.84 as the sp. gr. referred to turpentine. Multiply this by .87, the sp. gr. of the turpentine, and we get 1.6 as the true sp. gr. of sugar. For liquids we use the *specific-gravity flask* (Fig. 2), which is made and marked to contain a certain weight of water. Fill the flask with the liquid to be investigated and weigh it. Deduct the weight of the flask and divide this result by the weight of water the flask will hold. In practice the *hydrometer* is generally used. This is a hollow glass float with a graduated neck at its upper end, which indicates the specific gravity by the depth to which it sinks in the liquid. The urinometer [the illustration of the urinometer is in Part III, on the urine] is a hydrometer whose scale is constructed to measure the specific gravity of urine. For very accurate measurements of specific gravity the liquids must be at the standard temperature, which in this country is 60° F.

Fig. 2.

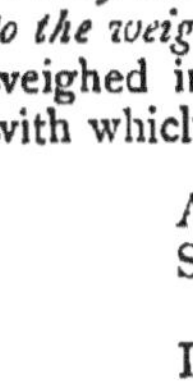

INTRODUCTION.

so rigidly as to give the body a definite shape; while in the liquid state the attraction is so slight as to allow the particles to move freely upon each other and the body to take the shape of the vessel that contains it. In the gaseous state the mutual attraction of the particles is entirely overcome, and their distance from each other depends upon the pressure to which the gas is subjected. The term fluid is applied to anything capable of flowing, whether liquid or gaseous. It is highly probable that all substances, which are not decomposed by heat or cold, are capable of existing in all three states. Heat is absorbed and cold produced wherever the particles are to be driven farther apart, as in the passage of a substance from the solid to the liquid or from the liquid to the gaseous state.

When the two solids, ice and common salt are mixed, they form a liquid, and great cold is produced.* Perspiration in evaporating assumes the gaseous state, and absorbs in the change so much heat that the body is kept at its normal temperature in spite of the hottest weather.†

On the other hand, when a substance passes from a rarer to a denser state it gives out again the heat absorbed in its passage in the opposite direction.

If we examine the infinite variety of substances upon our earth we find most of them are *compounds*, *i. e.*, they can be decomposed into two or more other substances, distinct in their properties from the substance from which they were derived and from each other. There are some substances which have never been decomposed. These are called *elements*. Only seventy elements are at present known; but, as our methods of investigation improve, this number may be increased by the discovery of other elements, or decreased by decomposing some of those now considered elements. Only about one-half of these enter into the materia medica, and will be noticed in this work.

---

* **Experiment.**—Fold tin-foil into the shape of a little dish; add powdered ice and salt. Spill water on the table and set the dish in it. Note how quickly it is frozen fast to the table.

† **Experiment.**—Put a little water in a similar dish. Against the sides and bottom throw a spray of ether. Note that the evaporation of the ether is so rapid that the water is quickly frozen.

TABLE OF ELEMENTARY BODIES, WITH THEIR SYMBOLS AND ATOMIC WEIGHTS.

(The more important are printed in capitals.)

Name.	Symbol	Atomic Weight	Name.	Symbol	Atomic Weight
ALUMINIUM,	Al	27	Molybdenum,	Mo	96
ANTIMONY (Stibium),	Sb	120	NICKEL,	Ni	58
ARSENIC,	As	75	Niobium,	Nb	94
BARIUM,	Ba	137	NITROGEN,	N	14
Beryllium,	Be	9	Norwegium,	Ng	214
BISMUTH,	Bi	208	Osmium,	Os	198
BORON,	B	11	OXYGEN,	O	16
BROMINE,	Br	80	Palladium,	Pd	106
CADMIUM	Cd	112	PHOSPHORUS,	P	31
Cæsium,	Cs	133	PLATINUM,	Pt	194.4
CALCIUM,	Ca	40	POTASSIUM (Kalium),	K	39.1
CARBON,	C	12	Rhodium,	Rh	104
CERIUM,	Ce	141	Rubidium,	Rb	85
CHLORINE,	Cl	35.5	Ruthenium,	Ru	104
CHROMIUM,	Cr	52	Samarium,	Sm	150
COBALT,	Co	59	Scandium,	Sc	44
COPPER (Cuprum),	Cu	63.4	Selenium,	Se	79
Didymium,	D	145	SILICON,	Si	28
Erbium,	E	166	SILVER (Argentum),	Ag	108
FLUORINE,	F	19	SODIUM (Natrium),	Na	23
Gallium,	Ga	70	STRONTIUM,	Sr	87.5
Germanium,	Ge	163	SULPHUR,	S	32
GOLD (Aurum),	Au	197	Tantalum,	Ta	182
HYDROGEN,	H	1	Tellurium,	Te	128
Indium,	In	113.4	Thallium,	Tl	204
IODINE,	I	127	Thorinum,	Th	231
Iridium,	Ir	192	TIN (Stannum),	Sn	118
IRON (Ferrum),	Fe	56	Titanium,	Ti	50
Lanthanum,	La	139	Tungsten, or Wolfram,	W	184
LEAD (Plumbum),	Pb	207	Uranium,	U	240
LITHIUM,	Li	7	Vanadium,	V	51.2
MAGNESIUM,	Mg	24	Ytterbium,	Yb	173
MANGANESE,	Mn	54	Yttrium,	Y	90
MERCURY (Hydrargyrum),	Hg	200	ZINC,	Zn	65
			Zirconium,	Zr	89.6

To explain the laws governing chemical phenomena we adopt the old *atomic theory.**

** Democritus, 460 B. C., said: "The atoms are invisible by reason of their smallness; indivisible by reason of their solidity; impenetrable and unalterable."

INTRODUCTION.

We will take up the theories and laws, not in the order of their enunciation, but of their natural sequence.

It is assumed that matter is composed ultimately of infinitely small particles called *atoms;* that each element is composed of *atoms*, all of a certain size, weight, etc. Atoms do not exist alone, but in groups called *molecules*. In an element the molecule is composed of pairs of atoms of the same kind; in compounds they consist of two or more atoms of different kinds. It has been determined that equal volumes of all substances in the gaseous state, and under like conditions, contain the same number of molecules. So a gallon of hydrogen gas and one of oxygen gas containing the same number of molecules, and those molecules consisting of pairs of atoms, must contain the same number of atoms. Furthermore, it is found that the gallon of oxygen is sixteen times as heavy as the gallon of hydrogen. So each oxygen atom must also be sixteen times as heavy as the hydrogen atom. Hydrogen being the lightest substance known, its *atomic weight* is taken as 1, and consequently the atomic weight of oxygen is 16. The atomic weights of other elements are determined in a similar way. By "atomic weight" is not meant the absolute weight of atoms (for that is not known), but the weight of the atom as compared to the hydrogen atom. The atomic weight of carbon is 12. If carbon combines with oxygen, atom for atom, the new substance (CO) resulting from that action will consist of molecules, in each of which the carbon will weigh 12 and the oxygen 16, and, as the whole mass is composed of these molecules, the same proportion obtains throughout the new compound. So 12 is found to be the *combining weight* of carbon, and 16 of oxygen. If, however, the combination should occur in the proportion of one atom of carbon to two atoms of oxygen, then each molecule must consist of 12 by weight of carbon to 32 of oxygen, and that must be the proportion throughout the entire substance.

Between these two compounds no intermediate one can occur, for the carbon atom must take one or two, or more, oxygen atoms. It cannot take a fraction of one, for atoms are indivisible. Hence, we deduce the following Law: *Substances combine in certain fixed proportions* (atomic weights), *or in multiples of these proportions.*

Symbols are abbreviations of the names of the elements. They consist of the initial letter of the Latin name; but if the names of several elements begin with the same letter, the single-letter symbol is reserved for the most common element, and for the others another letter is added. Thus, we have nine elements whose names begin with C; the most common is carbon, whose symbol is C; the others add other letters, as chlorine, Cl; cobalt, Co; copper (cuprum), Cu, etc. The symbol indicates just one atom. When more than one atom is to be represented, the number is written just after and below the symbol, thus, C_4.

Formulæ are to molecules what symbols are to elements. They indicate the kind and number of atoms composing the molecule. When more than one molecule is to be indicated, the number is placed in front of the formula, thus, $5H_2O$. A parenthesis inclosing several symbols or formulæ should be treated as a single symbol, thus, $2(NH_4)_2CO_3 = N_4H_{16}C_2O_6$.

An *equation* is a combination of formulæ and algebraic signs to indicate a chemical reaction and its results. As no matter is ever lost or created in a reaction, the number of each kind of atoms before the equality sign must be the same as after it.

PART I.—INORGANIC CHEMISTRY.

CLASSIFICATION OF THE ELEMENTS.—The elements are usually divided into two great classes: (*a*) *Metals*, about fifty-five in number, possessing a peculiar lustre, good conductors of heat and electricity, and whose oxides when combined with water form bases; (*b*) *Non-metals*, about fifteen in number, possessing little lustre, poor conductors of heat and electricity, and whose oxides combine with water to form acids. A better classification, and the one we shall adopt, is the following, based upon chemical properties:—

I. The **Hydrogen and Oxygen Group.**

II. The **Chlorine Group**: Fluorine, Chlorine, Bromine, Iodine.

III. The **Sulphur Group**: (Oxygen) Sulphur, Selenium, Tellurium.

IV. The **Nitrogen Group**: Nitrogen, Phosphorus, Arsenic, Antimony, Bismuth.

V. The **Carbon Group**: Carbon, Silicon, Tin and Lead.

VI. The **Alkaline Group**: Lithium, Ammonium, Sodium, Potassium, Rubidium and Cæsium.

VII. The **Alkaline Earths Group**: Magnesium, Calcium, Strontium, Barium.

VIII. The **Earths Group**: Boron, Aluminium, Lanthanum, Cerium, Didymium, etc.

IX. The **Zinc Group**: Zinc, Cadmium.

X. The **Iron Group**: Chromium, Manganese, Iron, Cobalt, Nickel.

XI. The **Copper Group**: Copper, Mercury.

XII. The **Silver Group**: Silver, Gold, Platinum.

I. Hydrogen and Oxygen Group.

In a strict arrangement hydrogen would be placed in Group I of the metals and oxygen in the sulphur group. But we will consider them in a group to themselves, because (*a*) of all the elements hydrogen is taken as the standard for atomic weights, combining weights, valence, etc.; (*b*) oxygen plays a most important rôle in chemistry, and its deportment with the other elements forms the basis of our classification; (*c*) the chemistry of these two will best serve as an introduction to the study of the other elements.

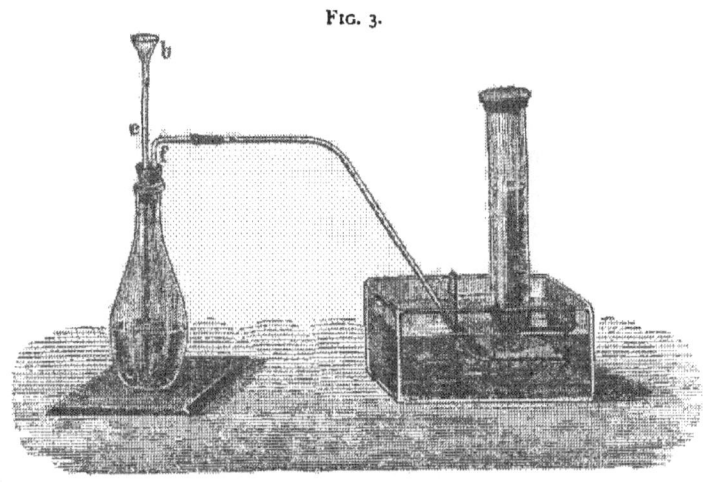

FIG. 3.

HYDROGEN ($H = 1$) *occurs* free in volcanoes, gas wells, etc.; combined in water and all organized bodies. All acids are salts of hydrogen. *Prepared* in various ways from its compounds,* the most convenient being to displace it from sulphuric acid by zinc, thus—

$$H_2SO_4 + Zn = ZnSO_4 + H_2.$$ (Fig. 3.)

Physical Properties.—Transparent, colorless, odorless, tasteless gas; the lightest substance known, fourteen and a half times as light as air; hence used in balloons. Long suspected to be a metal, because it displaces metals in chemical compounds, forms alloys with certain

---

* Experiment.—By means of a wire gauze spoon hold some sodium beneath the water and under a cylinder. The hydrogen gas liberated by the sodium from the water will rise in bubbles, fill the cylinder, and displace the water.

PART I.—INORGANIC CHEMISTRY.

metals, and conducts electricity. This was proved in 1877, when Pictet condensed it under great cold and enormous pressure into a bluish metallic liquid.

Chemical Properties.—Hydrogen does not support ordinary combustion or animal respiration. It burns in air with a pale but very hot flame.*† With pure oxygen it forms the oxyhydrogen flame. This is the hottest flame known, and a stick of lime held in it glows with dazzling brilliancy, forming the calcium or Drummond light. Mixed with air or oxygen, it explodes violently on contact with a spark.‡

FIG. 4.

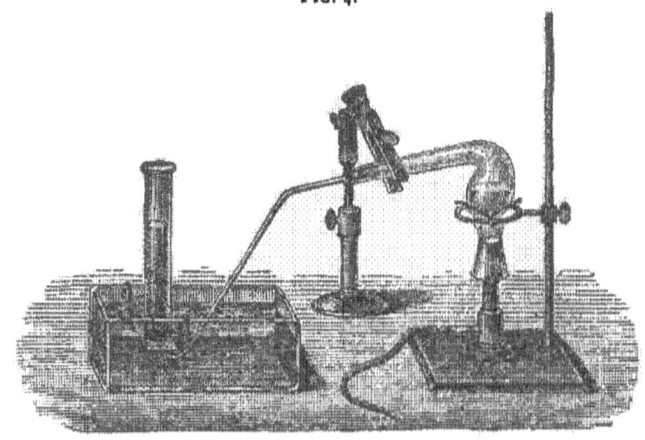

OXYGEN (O—16).—*Sources.* Most abundant of the elements, comprising one-fifth of the air, eight-ninths of water, one-half of the crust of the earth, and three-fourths of all organized bodies. *Prepared* most easily by heating potassium chlorate (Fig. 4):—

$$KClO_3 = KCl + O_3.$$

---

* **Experiment.**—If an inverted jar of the gas is suddenly turned up, and a flame held a foot or two above, the gas escaping from the jar rises rapidly, and in coming in contact with the flame burns with a slight explosion.

† **Experiment.**—If a jar of the gas be held mouth down and a candle be passed up into it, the gas ignites and burns quietly at the open end, while the candle passed up into the gas is extinguished, but may be relighted again by the burning gas as it is withdrawn.

‡ **Experiment.**—Fill a bladder or rubber bag with two parts of hydrogen and one of oxygen or five of air. Attach a tube and blow up soap bubbles in a basin. Touched with a flame, they explode.

If manganese dioxide (MnO_2) be mixed with the chlorate, the gas is liberated more quietly and at a lower temperature. The manganese dioxide is unaltered in the reaction. It seems to act by its mere presence, an influence called *catalysis*.

Physical Properties.—Gas; liquefied (Pictet, 1877) by great cold and intense pressure; colorless, odorless, tasteless; 1.10 times as heavy as air. Water dissolves only three volumes to the hundred, but enough to sustain aquatic life.

Chemical Properties.—Intense affinities; combines with every element except fluorine. The product of its action is called an *oxide*, and the process *oxidation*. Oxidation so rapid as to produce heat and light is called *combustion;* if no light, *slow combustion*. Substances that burn in air burn more brilliantly in oxygen,* and many substances that do not burn in air will burn in this gas.† By this property oxygen is usually recognized and distinguished from most other gases. Oxygen, especially in its diluted form (air), is the great supporter of combustion, for which its abundance and universal presence eminently fit it. Combustible and supporter of combustion are only relative terms. When a combustible substance burns in a supporter of combustion the union is mutual, one being as much a party to the action as the other. A jet of air ‡ or oxygen burns as readily in coal gas as a jet of coal gas burns in air or oxygen. The

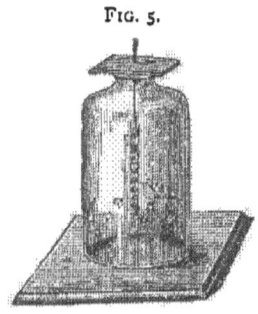

Fig. 5.

---

* **Experiment.**—A bit of phosphorus, dried by pressing between folds of blotting paper, is placed in a combustion spoon, ignited, and lowered into a jar of oxygen. The combustion is so intense that the phosphorus volatilizes, and its vapor burns throughout the jar with a brilliancy so dazzling that it is called the "phosphorus sun."

† **Experiment.**—A watch-spring is wound into a spiral, tipped with a bit of tinder or a piece of yarn dipped in sulphur. This is lighted and lowered into a jar of oxygen. (Fig. 5.) The iron catches fire and burns with brilliant scintillations, globules of melted iron falling and melting into the glass, unless the bottom be covered with sand or water.

‡ **Experiment.**—Secure an ordinary lamp chimney (Fig. 6) and a wide cork to fit its lower end. Pass through the cork a narrow tube (*a*) connected by rubber hose with the house gas, and a wider one opening into the air. Turn

one in greatest abundance is usually called the supporter of combustion.

Oxidizing agents are compounds in which oxygen is held so feebly it is readily given up to substances having greater affinity for it.

Uses.—The process of respiration is a species of combustion, and, as oxygen is the best supporter of combustion, it is the best (and only) supporter of animal respiration. Administered in capillary bronchitis, œdema glottidis, etc., when the patient cannot take in a volume of air sufficient to supply the requisite amount of oxygen.

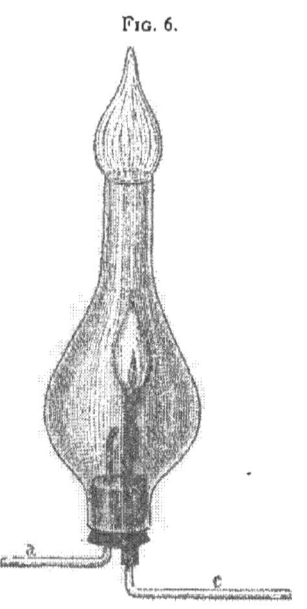

Fig. 6.

OZONE.—If through a portion of air or oxygen electric sparks be passed,* a part of the oxygen will acquire a pungent odor and peculiar properties. The same change may be induced by various chemical processes, *e. g.* by mixing permanganate of potassium and sulphuric acid, or when phosphorus partially covered with water is exposed to the air. This modified oxygen is called *ozone.* It is one and a half times as heavy as ordinary oxygen, for its molecule contains three instead of two atoms. Very energetic, oxidizing substances unaffected by ordinary oxygen. Oxidizes potassium iodide with

---

on the coal gas and light it as it issues from the tube. The cork with the flame (not too large) is then inserted into the chimney, where it continues to burn, sufficient air entering through the wide tube (*c*). Upon turning on more gas the air is crowded out and the chimney filled with coal gas. The gas flame disappears from the tube (*a*), and an air flame appears upon the tube (*c*) as the entering air burns in the atmosphere of coal gas. The excess of coal gas may also be lighted as it escapes, showing a gas flame above and an air flame within the chimney. On lessening the flow of gas the air will again be in excess, and the flame again appear on the narrow tube (*a*). In the gas flame above the lamp chimney (Fig. 6) heat some potassium chlorate in a combustion spoon until it melts and oxygen begins to bubble up. Then lower it into the atmosphere of coal gas within the chimney. The escaping oxygen burns brilliantly, the coal gas being the supporter of the combustion.

* Siemens' apparatus for ozoning oxygen (Fig. 7) consists of two tubes, the inner surface of the inner and the outer surface of the outer tube being coated

liberation of iodine, hence its *test:* paper dipped in a solution of potassium iodide and starch is colored blue in the presence of ozone.* Ozone is found in the air, especially after thunder-storms, and when present in considerable amount (as much as .00005 per cent.) is apt to irritate the respiratory tract; but by oxidizing infecting germs, etc., it prevents the spread of infectious diseases.

COMPOUNDS OF HYDROGEN WITH OXYGEN.—Two are known— hydrogen oxide, or water, H_2O; hydrogen peroxide, or oxygenated water, H_2O_2.

WATER (H_2O) *occurs* widely distributed in nature; an important

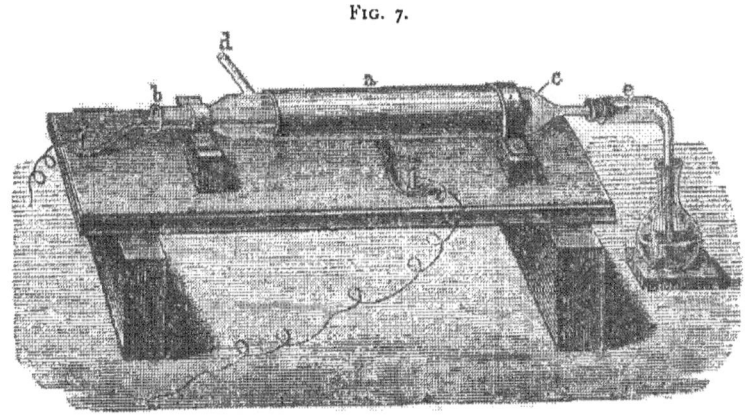

FIG. 7.

constituent of all organized tissues; forms seven-eighths of the human body.

Physical Properties.—Transparent, colorless, odorless, tasteless— liquid. Below 32° F. (0° C.) it is a solid (ice), and above 212° F. (100° C.) a vapor (steam or water gas). In solidifying, water expands; so ice floats. The boiling-point is higher than 212° F. under increased pressure or when it contains solid matter in solution.

---

with tin-foil, and each connected with the poles of an induction coil or Toepler-Holtz machine. A current of oxygen passing between these tubes may be ozonized to the extent of fifteen or twenty per cent.

* **Experiment.**—Pour a little ether into a beaker, across the top of which is a glass rod supporting a strip of blue litmus paper and one of paper dipped

PART I.—INORGANIC CHEMISTRY.

Water is the greatest of all solvents. The watery solution of a fixed substance is called a "*liquor*," and of a volatile substance an "*aqua*."

One body is said to dissolve in another when they coalesce and their particles intimately mingle. This is possible only in the liquid and gaseous states. When a substance dissolves it takes on the physical state of the solvent, *e. g.*, a solid or gas dissolving in water becomes a liquid and then mixes with the water, the gas elevating the temperature and the solid lowering it. Heat assisting the liquefaction of a solid, and opposing that of a gas, hastens the solution of the one and retards that of the other. Most solid substances when separating from a solution take with them, as a necessary part of the crystal, a certain definite amount of water—*water of crystallization*. This water does not modify the chemical nature of the substance, but is necessary for maintaining the crystalline form. If the crystal loses its water of crystallization by heat or exposure, it *effloresces* into an amorphous powder. Some substances when exposed absorb water from the air and *deliquesce* (melt down).

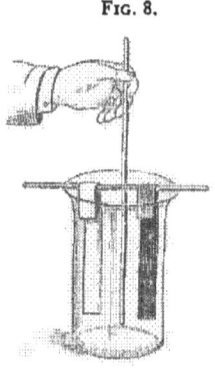

FIG. 8.

Chemical Properties.—The chemical composition of water may be proved by (*synthesis*) combining its constituents ($H_2 + O = H_2O$) * or by (*analysis*) passing the galvanic current through water until it is decomposed into its component gases ($H_2O = H_2 + O$). † Neutral in reaction ; combines with the oxides of the metals to form hydrates (bases), and with the oxides of the non-metals to form acids.

Natural waters are never pure. The nature of the impurities in

---

in potassium iodide and starch-water. Hold a hot glass rod in the jar (Fig. 8) ; the ether will undergo slow combustion, producing acid fumes which redden the litmus, and ozone which blues the other paper.

* A mixture of two volumes of hydrogen and one of oxygen exploded in a eudiometer (Fig. 9), produces only water.

† Fill the apparatus shown in Fig. 10 with water acidulated with sulphuric acid. Connect with a battery. The electricity passing through the water decomposes it into two volumes of hydrogen which collects in one tube and one volume of oxygen in the other.

water depends on the condition of the atmosphere through which it has fallen as rain, and the nature of the geological strata through or over which it has passed, for water dissolves something from almost everything it touches. Good, potable (drinkable) water should be cool, clear and odorless. It should contain just enough dissolved gases and solids to give it an agreeable taste, neither flat, salty, nor sweetish; and should dissolve soap without forming a curd. Water impregnated

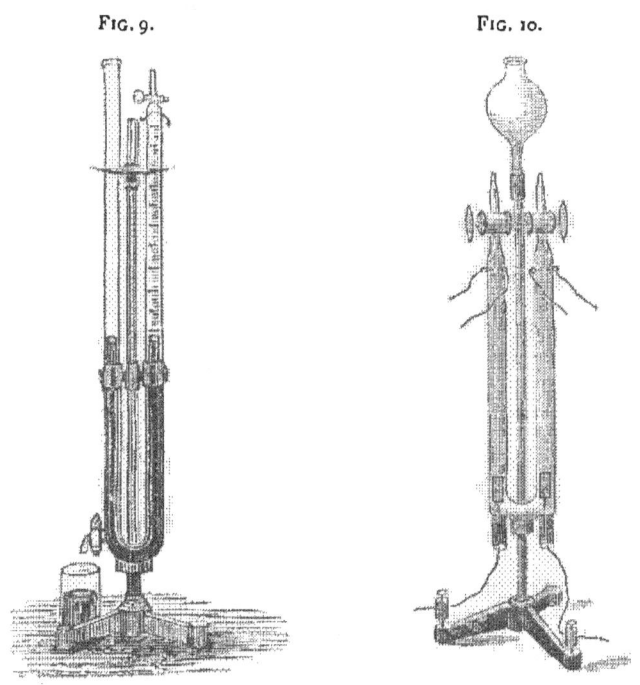

FIG. 9.   FIG. 10.

with inorganic matters, especially salts of calcium, is called hard. A much more serious contamination is with organic (animal and vegetable) matters. Such water is a prolific source of diease. It is probable, in fact almost proven, that most infectious diseases are due to microörganisms, many of which find the most favorable conditions for their life and growth in water contaminated with organic, especially animal, matter. Though chemical analysis cannot detect the disease-producing elements, it can detect organic impurity, without which they cannot exist. This is easily done thus: (1) Half fill a clean bottle with the water, warm, agitate, and critically smell it. A foul odor indicates organic impurity. (2) Fill a clean pint bottle three-fourths full, add a teaspoonful of the purest white sugar or gelatin; set aside in a warm place for two days, when, if it becomes cloudy (bacteria), it is unfit to use. These rough-and-ready tests are those best suited to the practitioner, the more exact methods being practicable only to the chemist.

To *purify* natural waters, they may be boiled to kill living organisms, and filtered to remove suspended matters; but for chemical

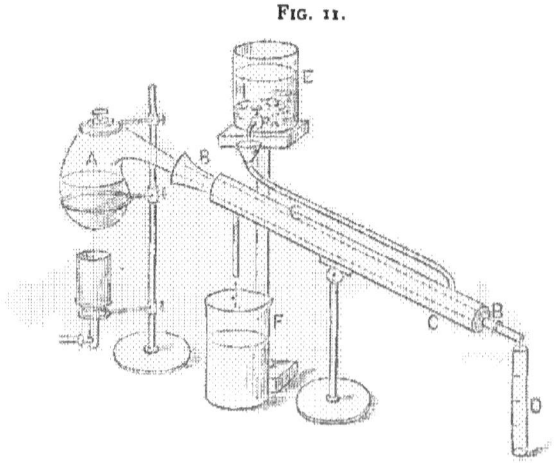

FIG. 11.

purposes, where great purity is desired, they are distilled * (*aqua destillata*, U. S. P.).

Mineral waters are those possessing special therapeutic value. They may be classed as follows:—

1. *Carbonated*, those charged with carbonic acid.

---

* When a liquid is rapidly vaporized, and the vapor, passing through a colder vessel, is recondensed, the process is called *distillation* (Fig. 11). If a solid be similarly treated it is called *sublimation*. When water containing solid matter in solution is distilled, the solids remain in the vessel, while the water passes over, enabling us to obtain perfectly pure water. When a mixture of two or more liquids is heated, the one having the lowest boiling-point distills first, leaving the others behind. This is called *fractional distillation*.

2. *Sulphur*, containing H_2S or some soluble sulphide.
3. *Alkaline*, containing alkaline salts of potassium, sodium, or lithium.
4. *Saline*, containing neutral salts.
5. *Chalybeate*, containing iron.
6. *Thermal*, or hot waters.

HYDROGEN DIOXIDE—*Oxygenated Water* (H_2O_2).—*Prepared* most easily diluted by passing CO_2 through water holding barium dioxide in suspension.

$$BaO_2 + CO_2 + H_2O = BaCO_3 + H_2O_2.$$

The $BaCO_3$ may be allowed to subside and the clear solution poured off.

Properties.—When concentrated it is a colorless, syrupy liquid, with a pungent odor and taste—prone to decompose into $H_2O + O$.

Used to bleach* the hair and skin, converting brunettes into blondes; as a disinfectant to ulcers, ozæna, and in diphtheria, especially when the membrane has invaded the nose; also as a test for pus in urine, with which it causes an effervescence.

The so-called "ozonized ether" used in the guaiacum test for blood is a mixture of hydrogen peroxide and ether.

RADICALS.—Every molecule is composed of two parts, called *radicals*, held together by chemical affinity. Both radicals may be elements, as in $H - Cl$, or one may be elementary and the other compound, as $H - NO_3$, or both compound, as $NH_4 - NO_3$. Some compound radicals can be isolated, *e. g.* by heat, $Hg - CN = Hg + CN$. Others decompose whenever set free. Whenever a galvanic current is passed through a compound, the chemical affinity is overcome by the electricity, and the molecule separates into its two radicals, one of which goes to the positive and the other to the negative pole.† Unlike electrical conditions attract, so the radical

---

* Experiment.—Secure an old oil painting darkened with age, or take paper dipped in lead acetate and blackened by hydrogen sulphide: wash it with hydrogen dioxide, and the dark stain will be made white by the lead sulphide being oxidized into sulphate.

† Experiment.—Into a jar put some water; add solutions of red litmus, potassium iodide, and boiled starch; connect with the galvanic battery. The electric current decomposes the potassium iodide into *iodine*, which gathers at the positive pole, producing a blue color, with the starch, and *potassium* at the negative, where it produces alkali, turning the red litmus blue.

going to the negative pole must be *electro-positive*, and the one going to the positive pole *electro-negative*. The metallic radicals are usually electro-positive and the non-metallic electro-negative.

Some radicals are more intensely electro-negative or electro-positive than others. In the following list the more common elements are so arranged that each is usually positive to those following it and negative to those preceding:—

Positive end: $+$ K, Na, Mg, Zn, Fe, Al, Pb, Sn, Bi, Cu, Ag, Hg,
Pt, Au, H, Sb, As, C, P, S, N, I, Br, Cl, F, O —Negative end.

A radical is electro-positive or electro-negative only in its relation to other radicals; for, while C is positive to O, it is negative to K.

In formulæ the electro-positive radical is written first and the electro-negative next.

The greater the difference between the electrical condition of two radicals, the greater the energy with which they unite and the more stable the product, and, *vice versâ; e. g.*, O has a strong affinity for K, a weak one for Cl, and will not unite with F under any circumstances. An idea once prevailed that the relations of affinities were fixed and constant between the same substances, and great pains were taken to construct tables similar to the above to show what was called the "precedence of chemical affinities." These tables showed the order of affinities for the circumstances under which the experiments were made, and nothing else.

The circumstances attending chemical reactions are so complicated that in the greater number of cases it is impossible to predict the precedence of affinities and the result of an untried experiment.

Among these modifying causes may be mentioned:—

1. *Temperature*, changes of which often reverse chemical affinities. Moderately heated, mercury and oxygen will readily combine, but when highly heated their affinity is destroyed, and they will refuse to unite, or, if already combined, will separate.

Ordinarily free carbon has no affinity for oxygen, but at high temperatures it surpasses all other elements in its greediness for that substance, even taking it from a metal so extremely electro-positive as potassium.

2. *Volatility.—Whenever in a mixture of two or more substances it is possible, by a rearrangement of the radicals, to form a compound*

volatile at the temperature of the experiment, such rearrangement will occur and the volatile compound be formed. For example:—

$$Fe\,S + H_2\,SO_4 = Fe\,SO_4 + H_2\,S;\ or,$$
$$2\,NH_4\,Cl + Ca\,CO_3 = (NH_4)_2CO_3 + Ca\,Cl_2;\ or,$$
$$H_3BO_3 + 3\,Na\,Cl = 3\,H\,Cl + Na_3\,BO_3.$$

3. *Insolubility.*—*Whenever, on mixing two or more substances in solution, it is possible, by rearrangement of the radicals, to form an insoluble compound, that rearrangement will occur and the insoluble compound be formed as a precipitate.* For example:—

$$Ca\,Cl_2 + (NH_4)_2\,CO_3 = Ca\,CO_3 + 2\,NH_4\,Cl.$$

It is especially important to remember this law, for its application in tests, incompatibilities, and antidotes.

4. *Nascent State.*—Ordinarily the atoms of an element are grouped in pairs, and hence somewhat indifferent to the attractions of other atoms; but just as they are being liberated (born) from a compound they are alone. Each atom, having no fellow, readily enters into combination with any atom it meets. This state is called *nascent* (*nasci*, to be born).

5. *Catalysis.*—This is the name given to the unexplained influence exerted by some substances of inducing chemical reactions between other substances without itself undergoing any change.

The valence of a radical is its combining value, or its value in exchange for other radicals.* Here again hydrogen is taken as the standard. A radical that combines with or takes the place of one atom of hydrogen is said to be *univalent* (one valued); of two atoms, *bivalent;* three, *trivalent;* four, *quadrivalent;* five, *quinquivalent;* six, *sexivalent.* The valence is indicated by a Roman numeral just above and after the radical, thus: (NH_4^I), Ca^{II}, $(PO_4)^{III}$, Si^{IV}, As^V, S^{VI}. The two radicals of every saturated compound must possess an equal number of unsatisfied valences. Hence,

In HCl the radical Cl is equivalent to 1 atom of hydrogen;
In H_2O the radical O is equivalent to 2 atoms of hydrogen;
In NH_3 the radical N is equivalent to 3 atoms of hydrogen;
In CH_4 the radical C is equivalent to 4 atoms of hydrogen.

---

* The student should bear in mind that valence has nothing to do with the combining weight or the chemical activity of an element.

Therefore Cl is univalent, O bivalent, N trivalent, and C quadrivalent.

The same regard for valence is observed when radicals are made to displace each other, thus: $H'_2(SO_4)^{II}$ requires two atoms of K^1 or one of Zn^{II} to form $K^1_2(SO_4)^{II}$ or $Zn^{II}(SO_4)^{II}$.

Some elements exercise more than one valence: *e.g.*, mercury may be univalent, as in HgI, or bivalent, as in HgI_2; or iron may be bivalent, as in $FeCl_2$, or the double atom (Fe_2) sexivalent, as in Fe_2Cl_6. The termination "*ous*" is given to those compounds in which the positive element exercises its lower valence, and "*ic*" to those in which the higher valence is exercised, as, $FeCl_2$, ferrous chloride; and Fe_2Cl_6, ferric chloride.

In the following table the most commonly occurring simple or elementary radicals are arranged according to their valence:—

TABLE OF VALENCE.

I	II	III	IV	V	VI
F, Cl	Ba, Sr	Al	C, Si	...	...
Br, I	Ca, Mg	Au	Pt	...	...
H, Ag	Cd, Zn	Bo	...	...	...
...	O	...	...	...	...
K, Na	Pb, Sn	...	Pb, Sn	...	...
(NH_4), Li	S, Se	...	...	...	S, Se
...	Fe, Cr	...	...	...	Fe_2, Cr_2
...	Mn, Co	...	...	...	Mn_2, Co_2
...	Ni	...	...	...	Ni_2
...	...	N, P	...	N, P	...
...	...	Bi, Sb, As	...	Bi, Sb, As	...
Cu, Hg	Cu, Hg	...	...	...	...

The next table shows the valences, together with the symbols and formulæ, of the most common electro-negative (acidulous) radicals:—

Univalent Radicals.
- Cl is the negative radical of all chlorides.
- Br is the negative radical of all bromides.
- I is the negative radical of all iodides.
- CN is the negative radical of all cyanides.
- HO is the negative radical of all hydrates.
- NO_3 is the negative radical of all nitrates.
- ClO_3 is the negative radical of all chlorates.
- $C_2H_3O_2$ is the negative radical of all acetates (Ac.).

Bivalent Radicals.
- O is the negative radical of all oxides.
- S is the negative radical of all sulphides.
- SO_3 is the negative radical of all sulphites.
- SO_4 is the negative radical of all sulphates.
- CO_3 is the negative radical of all carbonates.
- C_2O_4 is the negative radical of all oxalates (Ox.).
- $C_4H_4O_6$ is the negative radical of all tartrates (T.).

Trivalent Radicals.
- $C_6H_5O_7$ is the negative radical of all citrates (Cit.).
- PO_4 is the negative radical of all phosphates.
- BO_3 is the negative radical of all borates.

The student should learn these tables thoroughly, for with them he can easily know the formulæ of all the principal inorganic and organic compounds.

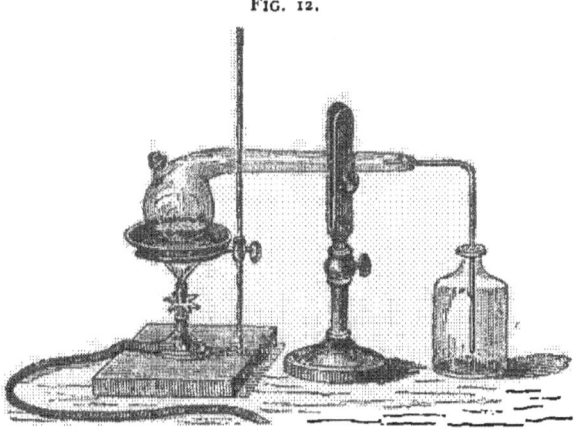

FIG. 12.

II. The Chlorine Group.

Name.	Derivation of Name.	Symbol.	At. Wt.
FLUORINE,	Fluor spar,	F,	19
CHLORINE,	χλωρός, green,	Cl,	35.5
BROMINE,	Βρῶμος, stink,	Br, .	80
IODINE,	Ἰώδης, violet,	I,	127

The members of this group are all univalent and much alike in their sources and physical and chemical properties. They differ in degree rather than in kind, forming a graded series. Hence we will consider them all together.

PART I.—INORGANIC CHEMISTRY.   29

Sources.—Never free in nature. The principal source of fluorine is fluor spar (CaF_2), while compounds of chlorine, bromine and iodine are abundant in sea and other salt waters.

Preparation.—Free fluorine is obtained only with great difficulty; the others may be prepared by removing the hydrogen from their hydrogen salts (hydracids) by means of oxygen derived from manganese dioxide, thus:—

$$4HCl + MnO_2 = MnCl_2 + 2H_2O + Cl_2.*$$
$$4HBr + MnO_2 = MnBr_2 + 2H_2O + Br_2.$$
$$4HI + MnO_2 = MnI_2 + 2H_2O + I_2.$$

Physical Properties.—Fluorine is a colorless gas, with properties resembling chlorine, but more intense. Chlorine is a very irritating yellowish-green gas, two and a half times as heavy as air, slightly soluble in water (three volumes), forming "*Aqua chlori*, U. S." Bromine is a red liquid, giving off red vapors of a disagreeable, irritating odor; very slightly soluble in water.

Iodine is a solid, in bluish-gray scales, which, when warmed, give off violet vapors; insoluble in water except by the intervention of an alkaline iodide; † soluble in alcohol; irritating, even caustic.

Chemical Properties.—Intensely electro-negative; great affinity for the metals, ‡ especially hydrogen. § In negativeness, and consequently in affinity for the metals, F is greatest, Cl next, Br next, and I least. Therefore, in compounds with the metals, F will displace

---

* Experiment.—Into a flask standing in a cup of sand over a heater (Fig. 12) pour several ounces of hydrochloric acid and half as much black oxide of manganese, and agitate. The gas passes out, and, being heavier than air, collects in the bottle, where its yellowish-green color makes it visible.

† Experiment.—To some water in a test-tube add a few scales of iodine; it does not dissolve. Now add a crystal of potassium iodide; it dissolves easily.

‡ Experiment.—Into a jar of chlorine introduce some copper or bronze foil, or sprinkle some powdered antimony. They inflame spontaneously.

§ Experiment.—(*a*) Into a jar of chlorine lower a lighted candle. The hydrogen of the tallow burns in the chlorine to form hydrochloric acid, and all the carbon is liberated as smoke. (*b*) Into a similar jar thrust a piece of paper dipped in warm turpentine. It inflames spontaneously and burns, evolving dense clouds of smoke.

Cl, and Cl will displace Br, and either F, Cl, or Br will displace I.*
These elements destroy coloring matters and noxious effluvia in two ways: (1) by abstracting their hydrogen; (2) by abstracting the hydrogen of water, setting free nascent oxygen, which oxidizes the matters in question.†

Medical.—Chlorine gas and bromine vapor are used for disinfection. Inhaled they cause severe coryza and bronchitis. Taken into the stomach, bromine and iodine cause gastro-enteritis. The antidote is boiled starch. Locally bromine is used as an escharotic and iodine as a counter-irritant.

Pharmaceutical.—The following preparations are officinal: *Tinctura Iodi* (℥j-Oj); and *Liquor Iodi Compositus* (Lugol's Solution) (Iodine ℨvj, potassium iodide ℥iss, and water Oj.) The so-called *colorless tincture of iodine* is made by adding ammonia-water to the tincture until it is decolorized by converting the iodine into ammonium iodide.

Tests.—In the free state chlorine and bromine may be known by their bleaching, color, odor, etc. Iodine is recognized by the blue color it strikes with starch.

NOTE.—ACIDS.—All acids have, as their (positive) basylous radical, hydrogen, which may be replaced by metals to form salts. They may generally be recognized by a sour taste and the property of turning vegetable blues (*e. g.*, litmus or purple cabbage) to reds. Acids whose acidulous (negative) radicals contain oxygen are called *oxacids;* those containing no oxygen, *hydracids.* The members of the chlorine group form both classes of acids.

---

* Experiment.—Take two large test-tubes half full of water. Into one put a grain of potassium bromide, into the other potassium iodide; add chlorine-water to each. The chlorine will liberate the bromine in one and the iodine in the other. This may be shown (*a*) by their color; (*b*) by adding a few drops of carbon bisulphide or chloroform, which on agitation will gather all the free bromine and iodine, and be colored brown with the one and violet with the other; (*c*) add a few drops of starch-water, which will give brown with bromine and a deep blue with iodine.

† Experiment.—(*a*) Into one bottle of chlorine gas introduce a piece of dry calico, into another a moist piece. The moist calico is rapidly bleached, while the dry is but slowly affected. (*b*) To a solution of indigo, cochineal, or some aniline color add chlorine-water. It is immediately decolorized.

PART I.—INORGANIC CHEMISTRY. 31

THE HYDRACIDS of the chlorine group are as follows:—

H + F = HF—Hydrogen Fluoride*—Hydrofluoric acid.
H + Cl = HCl—Hydrogen Chloride—Hydrochloric (muriatic) acid.
H + Br = HBr—Hydrogen Bromide—Hydrobromic acid.
H + I = HI—Hydrogen Iodide—Hydriodic acid.

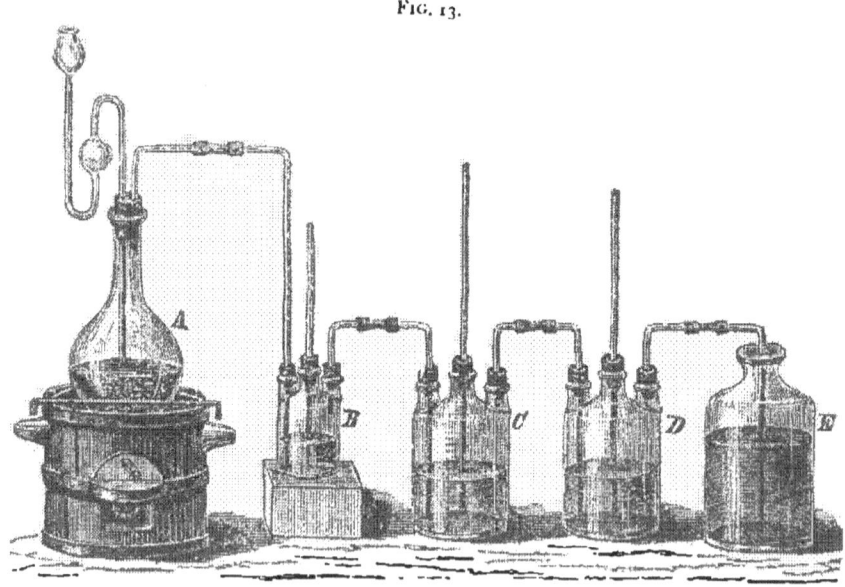

FIG. 13.

Prepared by treating the appropriate salt with H_2SO_4, thus:—

$CaF_2 + H_2SO_4 = CaSO_4 + 2HF.$
$2NaCl + H_2SO_4 = Na_2SO_4 + 2HCl.$†
$2KBr + H_2SO_4 = K_2SO_4 + 2HBr.$
$2KI + H_2SO_4 = K_2SO_4 + 2HI.$

---

* Binary compounds—*i. e.*, those of only two elements—are named by calling first the name of the positive and then that of the negative radical, affixing to the latter the termination "*ide.*"

† Experiment.—To prepare hydrochloric acid gas, put several ounces of common salt and about twice as much sulphuric acid into a flask, and warm. The gas comes off in abundance and may be collected in a dry bottle (like chlorine, Fig. 12), or over mercury. The solution of the gas (the ordinary form) is obtained by passing the gas through a series of Wolff bottles containing cold water and arranged as shown in Fig. 13.

Physical Properties.—Colorless, irritating gases; sharp, sour taste; very soluble, water dissolving several hundred times its own volume, forming *aqua* known by the simple name of the acid itself, thus: The officinal "hydrochloric acid" is a solution of the hydrochloric acid gas in water.

Chemical Properties.— Strong acids; true acids even without water.

Uses.—*HF* attacks silicon energetically, hence is used to etch glass; very poisonous, and burns made by it heal with difficulty.

HCl is very useful in the arts. *Aqua regia*, or nitro-muriatic acid, is a mixture of nitric and hydrochloric acids. It is the only solvent of gold and platinum. The metals are attacked by the nascent chlorine evolved by the oxidation of the H of the HCl by the O of the HNO_3. In medicine HCl is often prescribed as a tonic.

HBr, like all bromides, is a sedative. *HI*, like all iodides, is an alternative.

Tests.—Fluoride + H_2SO_4—etches glass.*

Chloride + $AgNO_3$—white precipitate, soluble in ammonia.

Bromide + $AgNO_3$—yellowish-white precipitate, slightly soluble in ammonia.

Iodide + $AgNO_3$—yellow precipitate, insoluble in ammonia.

If to a bromide or iodide some chlorine-water and starch paste be added, the bromine and iodine will be liberated, the bromine striking a brown and the latter a blue color with the starch.

OXACIDS are formed by oxides of non-metals combining with water. The elements of the chlorine group, being very negative, have but little affinity for oxygen. Iodine has most, bromine less, chlorine still less, and fluorine will not unite with oxygen at all.

Chlorine, bromine, and iodine each forms a series of oxides perfectly analogous, so we will notice only those of one—chlorine.

The several oxides are distinguished by prefixes derived from the

---

* *Experiment.*—On a plate of glass coated with wax or copper-plate varnish (six parts of mastic, one of asphalt, and one of wax dissolved in turpentine) draw a design with a pointed instrument. Invert over a lead dish and warm gently. Hydrofluoric acid gas is evolved and attacks the glass wherever the wax has been scratched off. Upon removing the wax the design is found permanently etched on the glass.

PART I.—INORGANIC CHEMISTRY.

Greek numerals indicating the number of oxygen atoms in the formula, thus:—

Cl_2O—Chlorine Monoxide.
Cl_2O_2 (?)—Chlorine Dioxide.
Cl_2O_3—Chlorine Trioxide.
Cl_2O_4—Chlorine Tetroxide.
Cl_2O_5—Chlorine Pentoxide.
Cl_2O_7—Chlorine Heptoxide.

These oxides combining with water form the corresponding acids, thus:—

$Cl_2O + H_2O = 2HClO$ —Hydrogen Hypochlorite—Hypochlorous acid.
$Cl_2O_3 + H_2O = 2HClO_2$—Hydrogen Chloride—Chlorous acid.
$Cl_2O_5 + H_2O = 2HClO_3$—Hydrogen Chlorate—Chloric acid.
$Cl_2O_7 + H_2O = 2HClO_4$—Hydrogen Perchlorate—Perchloric acid.

NOTE.—*The names of oxacids are derived from the **negative element** other than oxygen, and to this certain affixes and prefixes are added to indicate the degree of oxidation. The one containing more oxygen has the affix "-ic," less oxygen, " -ous." If there is in the same series another acid with more oxygen than the " -ic," it is given the prefix "per-;" if less than the " -ous," the prefix " hypo-" (under). Acids ending in "-ic" form salts ending in " -ate ;" those ending in "-ous" form salts ending in "-ite." The foregoing chlorine acids illustrate this.*

All these oxides, as well as their corresponding acids, are easily decomposed, sometimes with explosion; hence much used as oxidizing agents* and as explosive mixtures.† The most important of these salts is potassium chlorate, used in medicine and in the laboratory for the sake of its oxygen.

---

* Experiment.—Their oxidizing action on combustibles may be shown by: (*a*) Mix together a drachm each of powdered potassium chlorate and sugar; place on a brick and touch off with a glass rod dipped in sulphuric acid. A vigorous combustion occurs. (*b*) Drop some crystals of potassium chlorate into a conical glass of **water**; add several bits of phosphorus; then by means of a pipette introduce **sulphuric acid** at the bottom of the glass. The phosphorus takes fire and burns at the expense of the oxygen of the potassium chlorate.

† Experiment.—Mix on a sheet of paper a scruple of powdered potassium chlorate and five grains of some combustible powder, as sulphur, antimony sulphide, or tannin. Wrap it up in the paper, place upon an anvil, and strike with a hammer. It explodes violently.

III. **Sulphur Group.**

OXYGEN (already described), . O 16
SULPHUR, ... S 32
SELENIUM, ... Se 79.4
TELLURIUM, ... Te 128

The elements comprising this group are solid at ordinary temperatures; bivalent and sexivalent; possess electro-negative affinities

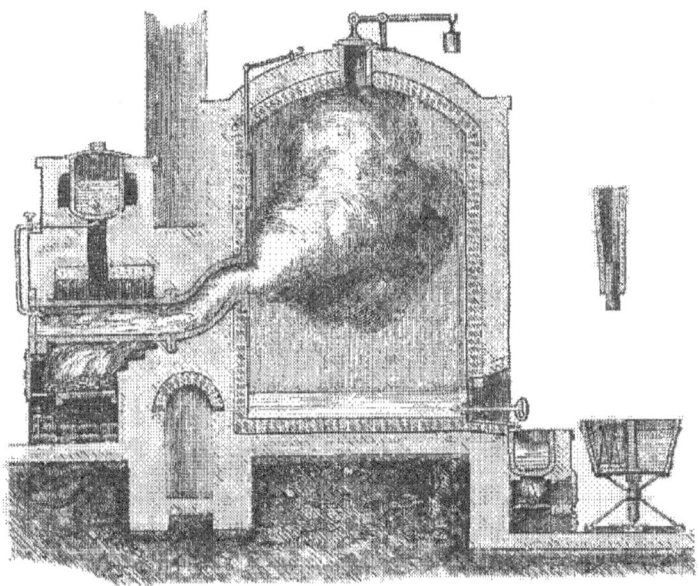

FIG. 14.

which, as in other groups, decrease as the atomic weights increase; form hydracids as well as oxacids.

The analogy between their compounds is shown in the following table:—

Hydro-ic Acid.	Dioxide.	Trioxide.	Hypo-ous Acid.	-ous Acid.	-ic Acid.
H_2S	SO_2	SO_3	H_2SO_2	H_2SO_3	H_2SO_4
H_2Se	SeO_2	SeO_3		H_2SeO_3	H_2SeO_4
H_2Te	TeO_2	TeO_3		H_2TeO_3	H_2TeO_4

Selenium and Tellurium are of no medical interest, and will not be further noticed.

PART I.—INORGANIC CHEMISTRY.

SULPHUR *occurs* free, especially in the neighborhood of volcanoes; occurs combined as sulphides and sulphates in many valuable ores, and in small quantity in the animal and vegetable kingdoms.

Preparation.—The native sulphur freed from stones is refined by distillation, as shown in Fig. 14. The crude sulphur is melted in the tank by the hot draft from the fire below, and then runs down through a pipe into the retort, where it is vaporized. This vapor, entering a large brick chamber, is condensed in fine, feathery crystals, called *flowers of sulphur* or *sublimed sulphur*. If the chamber be hot, it condenses into a liquid, which is drawn off and moulded into rolls, called *roll brimstone*. Sublimed sulphur is apt to contain more or less acid, and is washed (*sulphur lotum*). Boiled with lime and precipitated with HCl, it forms *sulphur precipitatum*, U. S. P. This mixed with water is *milk of sulphur* (*lac sulphuris*, U. S. P.).

Physical Properties.—A brittle yellow solid; insoluble in water, hence, tasteless, etc.

Chemical Properties.—Inflammable, hence called "brimstone" (burn-stone). Combines with metals,* forming sulphides.† Sulphur forms compounds remarkably analogous to those of oxygen, *e. g.* :—

H_2O . . . KHO . . . . CO_2 . . H_2CO_3 . . . . $HCNO$.
H_2S . . . KHS . . . . CS_2 . . . H_2CS_3 . . . . $HCNS$.

Uses.—In the arts, to make gunpowder, matches, etc.; in medicine, as a laxative, parasiticide, and alterative. We have only theoretical explanations of the method of its absorption; but that it is absorbed is certain, for persons taking it excrete enough to blacken silver carried on the person.

HYDROGEN SULPHIDE—H_2S—*Hydrosulphuric Acid or Sulphureted Hydrogen*—occurs in sewer gas and other effluvia from decomposing organic sulphurized matters, and in the water of sulphur springs.

Prepared in laboratory by decomposing a sulphide, thus :—

$$FeS + H_2SO_4 = FeSO_4 + H_2S.$$

---

* Experiment.—In a small glass flask, a little sulphur is heated to boiling. If now a bundle of fine copper wire or a piece of sodium, in a combustion spoon, be previously heated and then lowered into the vapor, it burns brilliantly.

† Experiment.—Mix in a dish equal parts of iron filings and flowers of sulphur: moisten with water and set aside. Within a half hour it gets hot, vaporizes the water, and is converted into a black mass of FeS.

Physical Properties.—Colorless gas, having the odor of rotten eggs or intestinal flatus; slightly soluble in water.

Chemical Properties.—Very feeble acid; burns with pale blue flame:—

$$H_2S + O_3 = SO_2 + H_2O.*$$

Forms characteristic precipitates with most metallic salts, hence a valuable test reagent.†

Tests.—The presence of H_2S even in minute quantities may be detected by its odor, and by its blackening paper moistened with a solution of lead acetate.

FIG. 15.

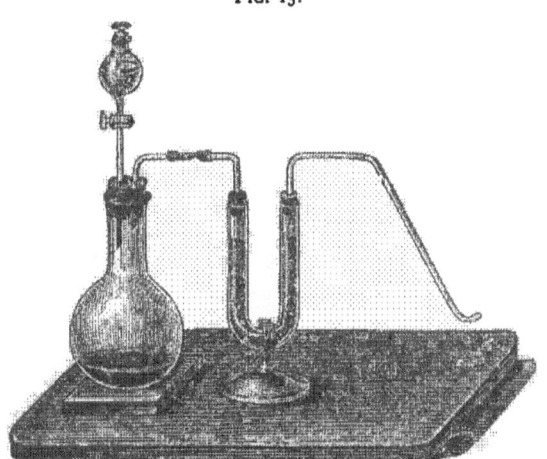

Preparation of H_2S.

Physiological.—When inhaled H_2S is an active poison, combining with the hemoglobulin and destroying its oxygen-carrying power. Even when highly diluted, as in the atmosphere of city dwellings,

---

* **Experiment.**—Burn the gas from a jet: (*a*) Hold near the flame a glass rod dipped in ammonia; white crystals of ammonium sulphite are formed. (*b*) Hold a cold, dry bell glass over the flame; it is bedewed with water.

† **Experiment.**—To show the action of H_2S on metallic salts, connect several wash bottles with the generator A, as shown in Fig. 16. A dilute solution of lead acetate is put in B, of tartar emetic (antimony) in C, of arsenic in D, of zinc sulphate in E. The gas in passing precipitates lead sulphide (black) in B, antimonious sulphide (orange) in C, arsenious sulphide (yellow) in D, zinc sulphide (white) in E.

clumsily "fitted with the modern conveniences," it produces a low febrile condition. When concentrated, or even moderately diluted (one per cent. and over), the gas proves rapidly fatal.

Treatment.—Fresh air, artificial respiration, and stimulation.

CARBON DISULPHIDE—CS_2.—Obtained by bringing S into contact with heated charcoal. A colorless, volatile liquid of a fetid odor, unless it is very pure. A valuable solvent for S, P, india-rubber, etc.

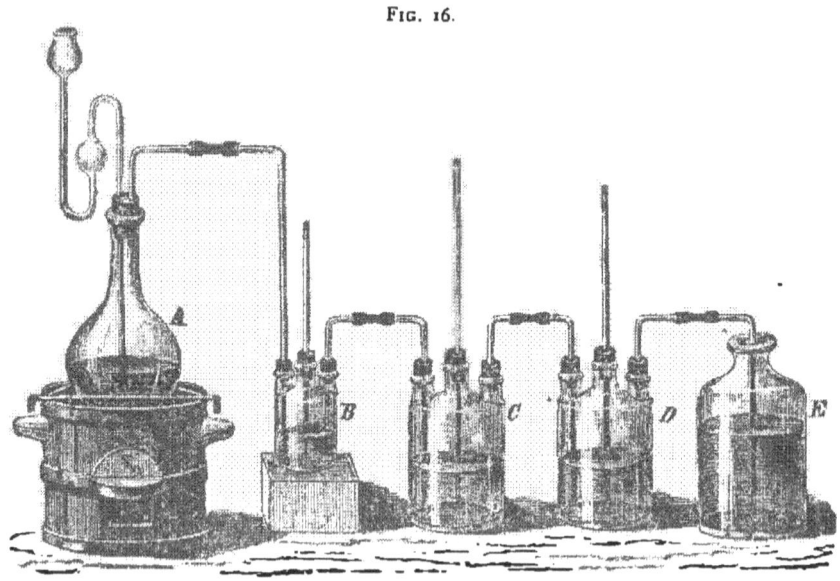

FIG. 16.

SULPHUR OXIDES AND ACIDS.

Dioxide—$SO_2 + H_2O = H_2SO_3$—Sulphurous acid.
Trioxide—$SO_3 + H_2O = H_2SO_4$—Sulphuric acid.

SULPHUR DIOXIDE, SO_2, *occurs* whenever sulphur or any of its compounds are burned in air or oxygen.

Prepared in laboratory by decomposing sulphuric acid by copper or charcoal, thus:—

$$2H_2SO_4 + Cu = CuSO_4 + 2H_2O + SO_2.$$
$$2H_2SO_4 + C = 2SO_2 + CO_2 + 2H_2O.$$

Physical Properties.—A colorless gas, with a suffocating odor (of burning matches); dissolves in water to form sulphurous acid (H_2SO_3).

Chemical Properties.—Neither burns nor supports combustion; a strong deoxidizer; by removing O from coloring matters and infecting germs it bleaches * and disinfects.

Uses.—Sulphur dioxide, sulphurous acid, and the sulphites possess the property of destroying microörganisms and arresting fermentations. A sulphite digested with sulphur forms a hyposulphite, thus:—

$$Na_2SO_3 + S = Na_2S_2O_3.$$

Sodium hyposulphite has the same uses as the sulphites, and is also a valuable solvent of the silver salts in photography.

SULPHUR TRIOXIDE, SO_3.—Made by oxidizing SO_2 in the manufacture of sulphuric acid. This is done upon a large scale by passing SO_2 from burning sulphur into a chamber kept filled with vapor of nitric acid, steam and air.† The nitric acid gives up a part of its oxygen to oxidize a portion of the SO_2 to SO_3.

$$2HNO_3 + 3SO_2 = 3SO_3 + H_2O + N_2O_2.$$

The SO_3 then combines with the water thus produced ($SO_3 + H_2O = H_2SO_4$), and more water is supplied by a jet of steam thrown constantly into the chamber.

The N_2O_2 has the power of taking up oxygen from the air and becoming N_2O_4.

$$N_2O_2 + O_2 = N_2O_4,$$

which in turn parts with this oxygen to oxidize a new quantity of SO_2.

$$N_2O_4 + 2SO_2 = N_2O_2 + 2SO_3.$$

Thus the process is kept up as long as the SO_2, air, steam, and N_2O_2

---

* **Experiment.**—Some sulphur is ignited beneath a tripod on which fresh flowers are placed, and the whole covered by a bell-glass. The flowers are bleached. The color may be restored by washing with some dilute alkali or acid that will combine with or displace the SO_2, or with very dilute nitric acid, which will restore the oxygen removed by the SO_2.

† The manufacture of sulphuric acid may be illustrated on the lecture table by the apparatus shown in Fig. 17. The lead chamber is represented by a large flask. Into this are led (*a*) N_2O_2 from the flask on the right; (*b*) SO_2 from a mixture of sulphur and manganese dioxide in the flask in the rear; (*c*) steam from the other flask, and (*d*) air or oxygen through the open tubes.

are supplied. The acid condenses with the water upon the floor of the chamber, and is drawn off, concentrated, and sold as

SULPHURIC ACID—H_2SO_4—"*Oil of Vitriol.*"

Physical Properties.—A dense, colorless, oily-looking liquid, without odor.

Chemical Properties.—Strong acid; very avid of water, not only dissolving in it, but combining with it, the act evolving considerable heat; chars organic matters by abstracting H and O to form water.*

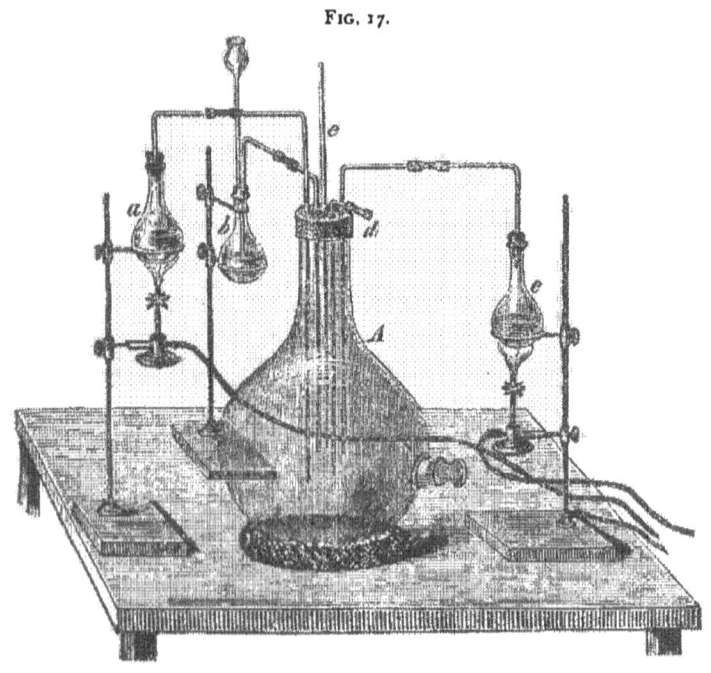

FIG. 17.

Uses.—So important in the arts that the commercial prosperity of a country may be measured by the amount of H_2SO_4 consumed. Properly diluted, it is a refrigerant tonic, but concentrated it is a severe caustic.

Tests.—(1) The concentrated acid, if placed on a piece of paper or

---

* **Experiment.**—Pour strong sulphuric acid on an equal quantity of sugar or strong syrup; the sugar is dehydrated and a mass of carbon left.

other organic material, will char it. If dilute, it will char the paper only after being warmed and concentrated by the evaporation of its water. (2) Sulphuric acid, or any other sulphate, will form with a solution of a barium salt a white precipitate ($BaSO_4$) insoluble in nitric or hydrochloric acid.

IV. Nitrogen Group.

NITROGEN,	N	14
PHOSPHORUS,	P	31
ARSENIC,	As	75
ANTIMONY (Stibium),	Sb	122
BISMUTH,	Bi	210

Trivalent and Quinquivalent.—This group, as shown below, forms a graded series from nitrogen and the negative to bismuth at the positive end:—

N	P	As	Sb	Bi
14	31	75	122	210
Gas, with full negative tendencies.	Sp. gr. 1.83. A soft solid. Easily volatilizable. Destitute of metallic lustre. Negative tendencies.	Sp. gr. 5.67. Solid. Volatilizable. Some metallic lustre. Both negative and positive tendencies.	Sp. gr. 6.7. Hard solid. Difficultly volatilizable. Great metallic lustre. More positive tendencies.	Sp. gr. 9.8. Very hard solid. Non-volatilizable. Full metallic lustre. Full positive tendencies.

The following will exhibit the relations of some of the most important compounds:—

Hydrides.	Chlorides.		Oxides.		Sulphides.	
	-ous.	*-ic.*	*-ous.*	*-ic.*	*-ous.*	*-ic.*
NH_3	NCl_3,	. .	N_2O_3,	N_2O_5	. .	. .
PH_3	PCl_3,	PCl_5	P_2O_3,	P_2O_5	P_2S_3,	P_2S_5
AsH_3	$AsCl_3$,	$AsCl_5$	As_2O_3,	As_2O_5	As_2S_3,	As_2S_5
SbH_3	$SbCl_3$,	$SbCl_5$	Sb_2O_3,	Sb_2O_5	Sb_2S_3,	Sb_2S_5
. .	$BiCl_3$,	. .	Bi_2O_3,	Bi_2O_5	. .	. .

NITROGEN *occurs* uncombined in the atmosphere; combined in some mineral and in all vegetable and animal bodies, especially in the more highly organized tissues.

Prepared most easily by burning phosphorus in a confined space

PART I.—INORGANIC CHEMISTRY. 41

until the oxygen is removed from the air.* Prepared in this way it contains small quantities of other gases found in air. To prepare it pure, heat ammonium nitrite ($NH_4NO_2 = 2H_2O + N_2$).

Physical Properties.—A colorless, tasteless, odorless gas, a little lighter than air.

Chemical Properties.—Little tendency to combine with other elements, and its compounds, once formed, are very prone to decom-

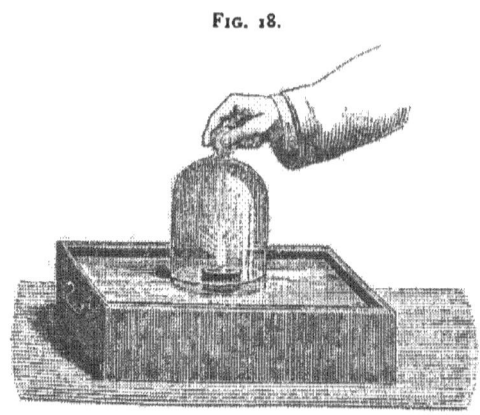

FIG. 18.

pose, either with violent decomposition † or gradual putrefaction ; neither combustible nor a supporter of combustion ; negatively poisonous.

THE ATMOSPHERE.—Air,‡ considered by the ancients one of the

---

* **Experiment.**—A flat piece of cork floating on water supports a capsule containing a bit of phosphorus carefully dried. This is ignited and immediately covered with a bell jar. The jar is filled with a dense white cloud from the combustion, which ceases only when the oxygen is all consumed. At first the air expands and some may be forced out. Upon cooling the water rises to take the place of the oxygen, and the white fumes gradually dissolve in the water, and the nitrogen is left clear and comparatively pure.

† **Experiment.**—To tincture of iodine add excess of ammonia water. Filter to separate the precipitated iodide of nitrogen. Put portions of this on separate bits of paper and set aside. When dry they explode on the slightest touch.

‡ Proofs that air is a mixture : (1) Its constituents are not in atomic proportions ; (2) air can be made by mechanically mixing the gases ; (3) solvents may remove one gas without affecting the others, each dissolving according to its own solubility.

four elements, is neither an element nor a compound. It is a mixture mainly of nitrogen and oxygen, the function of the former being to dilute the latter. Miller gives the average composition of air as follows:—

	Volumes.
Nitrogen,	77.95
Oxygen,	20.61
Carbon dioxide,	.04
Aqueous vapor,	1.40

Also traces of nitric acid, ammonia, sodium chloride, ozone, dust, bacteria, germs, etc. In the neighborhood of large cities various other substances are poured into the air from manufactories. Yet, owing to the rapid diffusion of gases, the composition of the air is almost the same everywhere.

Watery Vapor.—The higher the temperature the more water air will hold. A warm, dry air, when cooled, will appear damp, and the temperature at which it begins to deposit its water is its *dew-point*. A cold, damp air, when heated, becomes capable of holding more water, and appears dry; hence the necessity of supplying water to the heated air of our rooms in winter, especially in cases of bronchitis or catarrhal croup. Even in health a very dry air irritates the air-passages, produces dryness of the skin and *malaise;* while a very moist atmosphere retards evaporation from the skin and lungs, raises the body temperature, and becomes oppressive.

Suspended matters in air are of a great variety of substances. The irritation of dust incident to certain trades may cause chronic bronchitis, emphysema, and phthisis. Germs floating in the air are believed to be the cause of many contagious, infectious, and malarial diseases. The best disinfectants * are (*a*) free ventilation and consequent dilution; (*b*) chlorine, bromine, iodine, and sulphur dioxide.

NITROGEN HYDRIDE—AMMONIA, NH_3.—*Occurs* in the effluvia from decomposing nitrogenized organic bodies; for nitrogen and hydrogen unite only in the nascent state. (See page 26.) First obtained by distilling camel's dung, near the temple of Jupiter Ammon in Libya; hence called "ammonia." Obtained by heating clippings of hides,

---

* *Disinfectants* destroy the power to infect, whether it be due to germs or other agent. *Germicides* destroy **germs**. *Antiseptics* prevent putrefaction. *Antizymotics* prevent **fermentation**. *Deodorizers* destroy offensive odors.

PART I.—INORGANIC CHEMISTRY. 43

hoofs and horns,* especially of deer, in closed retorts (destructive distillation), it was called *spirit of hartshorn*. Coal contains about two per cent. of nitrogen, which in the manufacture of coal gas comes off as ammonia. In washing the coal gas the ammonia dissolves in the water. This *aqua* is its commercial source.

Prepared in laboratory by driving the ammonia off from the *aqua* by means of heat.

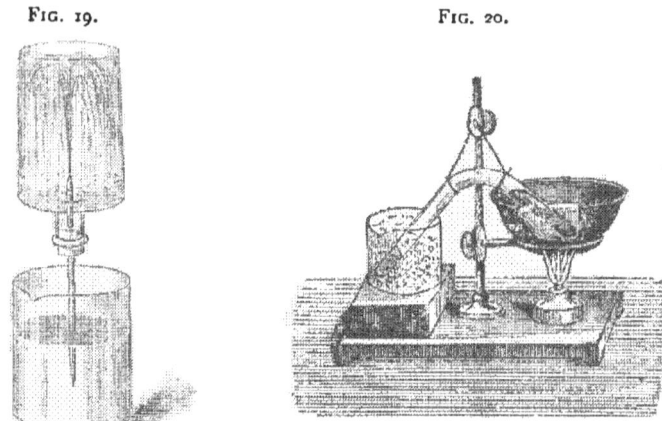

FIG. 19.   FIG. 20.

Physical Properties.—Transparent, colorless gas, of an irritating odor; condenses under a pressure of 6½ atmospheres into a colorless liquid;† very soluble in water, which dissolves from 500 to 1000 times its own volume.‡ Administered by inhalation as a stimulant

---

* Experiment.—Mix calcium, potassium, or sodium hydrate with some nitrogenous substance, as albumin or clippings of horn, hoofs, flannel or lean meat. Heat in a test-tube. Ammonia gas is evolved, recognized by its odor, alkalinity, or by white fumes forming when a glass rod moistened with HCl is thrust into the tube.

† Experiment.—Make ammonium silver chloride by passing ammonia gas over silver chloride. Enclose this in a bent tube (Fig. 20). The end containing the compound is heated in a water bath, while the other is cooled in an ice mixture. Ammonia gas is driven off from the compound, and condenses into a colorless liquid in the cold end of the tube.

‡ Experiment.—The absorption of ammonia gas by water may be illustrated by filling a large bottle with the gas by upward displacement and closing the mouth with a rubber cork through which passes a glass tube sealed at the outer end. If this sealed end be plunged under water and then broken off, the water rushes in, forming a fountain (Fig. 19). If the water be colored with red litmus solution it will become blue as it enters the bottle, showing the alkalinity of the solution.

in fainting fits, etc., but care must be taken, for its too liberal use may cause spasm of the glottis or induce a fatal bronchitis.

Tests.—(1) Smell; (2) white fumes with HCl; (3) turns moistened red litmus paper blue.

NITROGEN OXIDES.

    Monoxide—$N_2O + H_2O = 2HNO$ = Hyponitrous acid.
    Dioxide—N_2O_2. No corresponding acid.
    Trioxide—$N_2O_3 + H_2O = 2HNO_2$ = Nitrous acid.
    Tetroxide—N_2O_4. No corresponding acid.
    Pentoxide—$N_2O_5 + H_2O = 2HNO_3$ = Nitric acid.

FIG. 21.

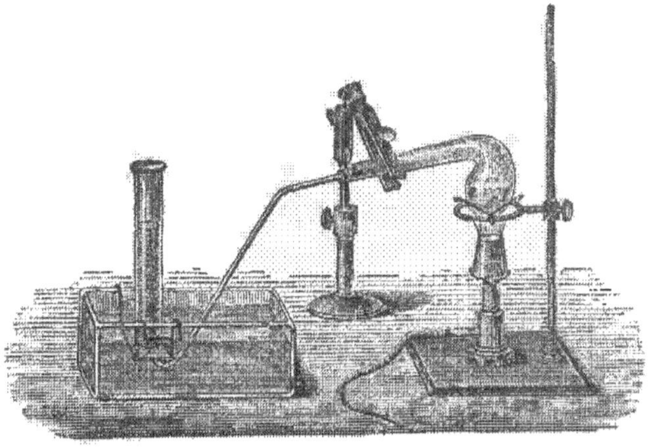

Making N_2O.

NITROGEN MONOXIDE—N_2O (*Nitrous Oxide—Laughing Gas*).— *Prepared* by heating ammonium nitrate, as shown in Fig. 21.

$$NH_4NO_3 = N_2O + 2H_2O.$$

Physical Properties.—Colorless, odorless gas, of sweetish taste. Dentists keep it liquefied under pressure in iron cylinders.

Chemical Properties.—By the ease with which it gives up its O it is a supporter of combustion and life, next to O itself.

Medical.—Inhaled, diluted with air, it produces exhilaration of spirits, muscular activity, and then complete anæsthesia. Used in dental and other brief minor operations.

NITROGEN DIOXIDE—N_2O_2 (*Nitric Oxide*).—*Prepared* by action of nitric acid on copper:—*

$$3Cu + 8HNO_3 = 3Cu(NO_3)_2 + 4H_2O + N_2O_2.$$

A colorless gas, which, when coming in contact with free O, forms red vapors of N_2O_3 and N_2O_4; hence a test for free O.

NITROGEN TRIOXIDE—N_2O_3 (*Nitrous Acid*—HNO_2).—Nitrous acid is known only in its salts, the nitrites. These are produced in nature by the oxidation of nitrogenous organic matter in the presence of certain forms of microscopic life.

This nitrification occurs in waters polluted with organic matter, and normally in the soil, where the acid so formed combines with bases. Hence nitrites in water is evidence of previous contamination with nitrogenous matter. Further oxidation forms nitrates.

NITROGEN TETROXIDE—N_2O_4—*occurs* in company with N_2O_3 in the brown fumes given off whenever nitric acid is decomposed, as in certain laboratory and manufacturing processes. *The effect* of breathing air thus contaminated is to produce chronic inflammation of the respiratory tract. If the vapor be more concentrated the effects are more acute and serious. At first there is only a cough, in two or three hours a difficulty of breathing, and in about twelve hours, death. The remedy is ventilation.

NITROGEN PENTOXIDE—N_2O_5—is of no medical interest.

NITRIC ACID—HNO_3 (*Aqua Fortis*)—*occurs* in traces in the atmosphere and as nitrates in the soil. (See Nitrites.)

Prepared by distilling a nitrate with sulphuric acid.

$$2KNO_3 + H_2SO_4 = K_2SO_4 + 2HNO_3.\dagger$$

---

* Experiment.—Copper turnings, clippings, or wires are placed in a flask, and nitric acid diluted with half its volume of water is poured in, and the flask set in cold water. Red fumes soon fill the flask, but when these have escaped the gas appears colorless, turning red, however, on reaching the air. The colorless gas is collected over water.

† Experiment.—In the laboratory nitric acid may be prepared with the apparatus shown in Fig. 22. Equal parts of sodium nitrate and sulphuric acid are heated in the retort. The nitric acid produced is vaporized by the heat and recondensed in a receiver kept cool by a wet cloth, over which flows a stream of water from an elevated vessel.

Physical Properties.—Heavy liquid, colorless, but if old and exposed to light it may be yellow or orange from presence of N_2O_3 and N_2O_4. Like all other nitrates, it is soluble in water.

Chemical Properties.—Energetic oxidizer;* corrosive; stains skin indelibly yellow.

Medical Uses.—The strong acid is an escharotic, coagulating the albumin of the tissues; the dilute, a refrigerant tonic.

Tests.—(1) Yellow stain. (2) Add H_2SO_4, and then a crystal of $FeSO_4$ dropped in will be colored brown if nitric acid or any nitrate be present.

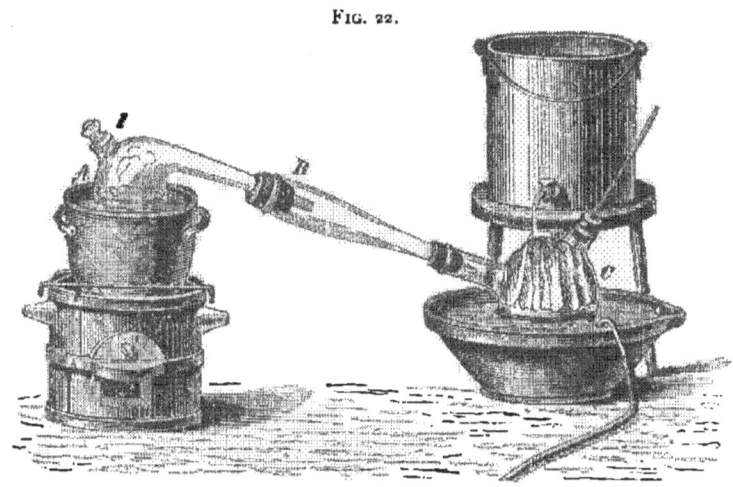

FIG. 22.

Making HNO_3.

PHOSPHORUS (Light-bearer) *occurs* combined with O in the ancient unstratified rocks. These disintegrate and form soil, from which the P passes into the organisms of plants, and thence into the bodies of animals. First isolated by Brandt (1669) from urine; now obtained from bones.

Physical Properties.—A soft, yellowish solid, resembling unbleached

---

* **Experiment.**—Into a mixture of strong sulphuric and nitric acids pour from a beaker tied to a long stick some warm turpentine. The oxidation is so rapid that the turpentine is inflamed.

wax.* Insoluble in water, but soluble in carbon disulphide, ether, chloroform, oils, etc.

Chemical Properties.—Very inflammable,† so kept under water; exposed to the air, it undergoes a slow combustion, emits the odor of ozone, and is luminous in the dark.

Physiological.—Liable to inflame from careless handling, and burns by it are difficult to heal. In medicinal doses, a nerve tonic and aphrodisiac; in larger quantities a virulent poison and gastro-irritant. Sometimes given with homicidal intent, but more frequently taken accidentally as rat poison, tips of matches, etc. Workmen in match factories suffer from irritation of stomach and bowels, caries of teeth, necrosis of bones, especially of lower jaw, and from fatty degeneration of various organs. This may be prevented by using the red allotropic variety, which is harmless.

No good antidote. Evacuate the stomach; give copper sulphate ‡ as emetic and antidote; give old turpentine, the ozone of which oxidizes the P. Avoid fats, for they dissolve it.

Tests.—(1) Shines in the dark; (2) emits garlicky odor.

PHOSPHORUS HYDRIDE.—PH_3 (*Phosphoretted Hydrogen—Phosphine*)—*occurs* mixed with other hydrides of P in the gases arising from decomposing animal or vegetable matters, especially under water; hence seen as the *ignis fatuus*, or "Will-o'-the-wisp," over marshes and graveyards.

Prepared by boiling phosphorus in a solution of caustic potash. §

---

* When heated to 500° F. in an atmosphere incapable of acting upon it, phosphorus is converted into a reddish-brown powder, which, unlike ordinary phosphorus, is not poisonous, not inflammable, and insoluble in the ordinary solvents.

† Experiment.—Dissolve some phosphorus in carbon disulphide. Pour this on a sheet of filter paper hung on a retort stand. Soon the solvent evaporates and leaves the phosphorus in such a fine state of division that it inflames spontaneously.

‡ Experiment.—Place a clean bit of phosphorus for a minute in a solution of copper sulphate. Remove, and note the coating of metallic copper.

§ Experiment.—Into a retort, whose delivery tube dips under water in a dish, add liquor potassæ and a few bits of phosphorus. Expel the air by passing hydrogen or illuminating gas through the retort, or by adding a few drops of ether, the vapor of which does the same thing. On applying heat the hydrogen or illuminating gas or ether vapor first escapes, then come bubbles of PH_3, each of which, as it bursts into the air, ignites spontaneously, forming beautiful rings of white smoke rotating on their circular axes. These may ascend to the ceiling if the air be still.

Properties.—Colorless gas, of a garlicky odor; inflames spontaneously upon coming in contact with the air; very poisonous.

PHOSPHORUS OXIDES. These are analogous to the oxides of hydrogen, and form, on the addition of water, analogous acids.

PHOSPHORUS PENTOXIDE (P_2O_5) is produced whenever P burns in

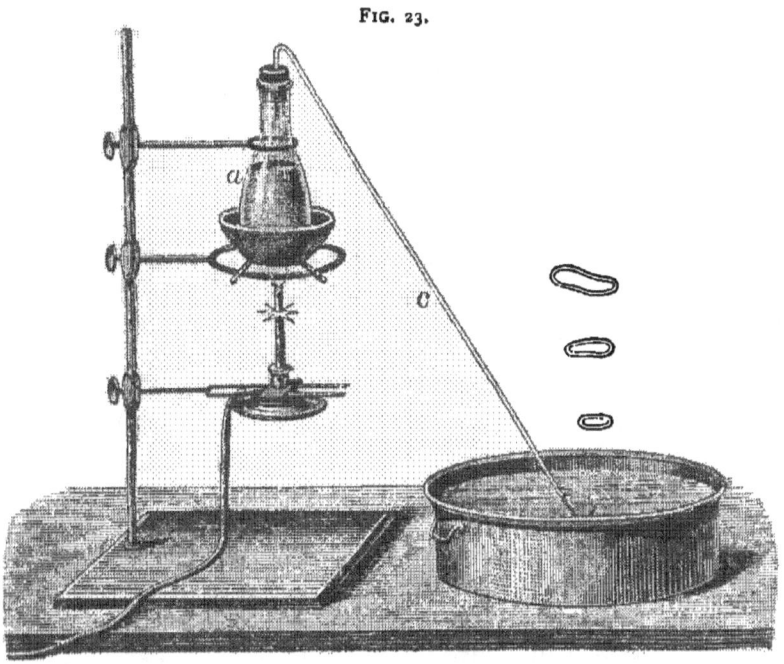

FIG. 23.

air* or O; and forms three different phosphoric acids by combining with one, two or three molecules of water, thus:—

$P_2O_5 + 3H_2O = H_6P_2O_8 = 2H_3PO_4 =$ Orthophosphoric acid.
$P_2O_5 + 2H_2O = H_4P_2O_7 =$ Pyrophosphoric acid.
$P_2O_5 + H_2O = H_2P_2O_6 = 2HPO_3 =$ Metaphosphoric acid.

ORTHOPHOSPHORIC ACID.—Never found free, but is widely dis-

---

* **Experiment.**—A little stand in the middle of a dinner-plate supports a capsule, into which is put a bit of phosphorus freed from adhering water. This is ignited and covered with a bell jar. This jar is filled with clouds of P_2O_5, which, aggregating, fall into the plate like a miniature snow-storm.

PART I.—INORGANIC CHEMISTRY. 49

seminated in the three kingdoms of nature in its salts, the phosphates. Being the phosphoric acid most used in medicine (the other two are poisonous), it is usually called simply "phosphoric acid." Transparent, odorless, colorless, syrupy liquid. Being tribasic, it forms three classes of phosphates by displacement of one, two, or three atoms of the basic hydrogen, thus:—

$$KH_2PO_4, K_2HPO_4, \text{ and } K_3PO_4.$$

In the diluted form (*acidum phosphoricum dilutum*) it is prescribed as a tonic, especially in dyspepsia.

Tests.—Add a few drops of the magnesian fluid ($MgSO_4$, NH_4Cl, and NH_4HO, each one part, water eight parts); a white precipitate indicates phosphoric acid or other phosphate.

ARSENIC *occurs* mostly as sulphide, usually associated with other metals. The ore is roasted, and the resulting oxide heated with carbon (charcoal) gives the metal. This is a brittle, steel-gray, crystalline solid, possessing a metallic lustre. Heated out of contact with air it sublimes; in air it burns with a bluish-white flame, emitting the odor of garlic and white clouds of As_2O_3. It combines with many elements; the metallic arsenides resemble alloys. *Used* in pyrotechny and in the manufacture of shot, pigments and fly-poison. All its compounds are poisonous.

ARSENIOUS HYDRIDE—AsH_3—*Arseniuretted Hydrogen—Arsine*— is of great practical interest to the toxicologist, as its formation constitutes one of the most delicate tests for arsenic. Forms whenever hydrogen is generated in presence of an arsenical compound.

ARSENIOUS IODIDE—AsI_3.—*Prepared* by fusing together atomic proportions of its constituent elements. It enters into *Donovan's Solution, liq. arsenii et hydrargyri iodidi*, U. S. P.

ARSENIOUS SULPHIDE—As_2S_3—*occurs* native as *orpiment*. *Prepared* by precipitating an arsenious compound with H_2S. Bright yellow powder, insoluble in water or acid solutions, but soluble in alkaline. Another sulphide is *realgar*, AsS_2. Both are *used* as pigments—the orpiment as a yellow, the realgar as a red.

OXIDES AND ACIDS.

$$As_2O_3 + 3H_2O = 2H_3AsO_3, \text{ (ortho) Arsenious acid.}$$
$$As_2O_5 + 3H_2O = 2H_3AsO_4, \text{ (ortho) Arsenic acid.}$$

ARSENIOUS OXIDE—As_2O_3. *Arsenic, White Arsenic, Ratsbane, Arsenious Acid.*—This is not only the most important compound of arsenic, but the most important of toxic agents, whether we consider the deadliness of its effects or the fatal frequency of its administration. When recently made it is in glassy lumps, which on exposure become crystalline and opaque. When sublimed it is deposited again in brilliant octahedral crystals. It is odorless, almost tasteless—slightly sweetish. When powdered arsenic is thrown upon water it does not all sink, notwithstanding its heaviness, but floats, showing a repulsion of the water. Very slightly soluble in water, even boiling water dissolving less than two per cent. If the water be made acid or alkaline, it dissolves more readily. When arsenic dissolves in water it forms *arsenious acid*, H_3AsO_3.

There are two officinal solutions, each containing one per cent. of arsenic: (1) *Liq. acidi arseniosi*, in which the water is acidulated with HCl; (2) *Fowler's Solution, liq. potassii arsenitis*, in which the water is made alkaline by K_2CO_3.

ARSENIC OXIDE.—*Arsenic pentoxide* is made when arsenious oxide (As_2O_3) is treated with an oxidizing agent, as nitric acid. It is quite soluble in water, with which it forms a series of *arsenic acids* (ortho-, pyro- and meta-) analogous to the phosphoric acids.

Toxicology of Arsenic.—The deadly effect of arsenical compounds has been known from remote antiquity, and they have probably been more used for homicidal purposes than all other toxic agents combined. Although chemistry has made its detection easy and certain, arsenic is so cheap, so readily administered to the unsuspecting victim, and so deadly, that it is still a favorite with the murderer. Owing to the extensive use of arsenical compounds as insect-powders (Paris green, etc.), and as pigments for wall-paper, toys, confectionery, etc., cases of accidental poisoning are quite common.

Few physicians have the training and facilities to undertake an extended analysis, but they should all know the simpler tests, so as to promptly recognize the nature of the poison and combat it intelligently and successfully. Besides, the physician, being early in the case, can by wise precautions prevent breaks in the chain of evidence; protecting the prisoner if innocent, and closing loop-holes of escape if guilty. If foul play is suspected, he should commit all his observations to writing, for notes to be admitted as evidence must be the original ones taken at the time. Having collected the urine,

PART I.—INORGANIC CHEMISTRY.   51

fæces, vomit, and the suspected vehicle of the poison, and having tested some or all of them to verify his suspicion, he should place them under seal or lock and key. He should carefully reserve his opinion, lest he do injustice to the innocent or warn the guilty. In case of death, the coroner should be notified and an autopsy held, in presence of the chemist if possible. The stomach and entire intestinal canal, ligated at both ends, half of the liver, the whole brain, spleen, one kidney, and any urine remaining in the bladder should be saved. These, if possible, should be preserved in separate jars, to which a little pure chloroform may be added to prevent decomposition. These jars must be new and clean, closed with new corks or glass—not zinc caps. They are then to be labeled, and also sealed and stamped, so they cannot be opened without detection, and as soon as possible turned over to the chemist or prosecuting officer.

The symptoms of arsenical poisoning are those common to all intense irritants, viz., nausea, vomiting, burning pain in the epigastrium, purging, cramps, thirst, fever, rapid pulse, etc., ending in collapse. Smallest fatal dose is two grains, and death usually occurs in twenty-four hours.

Treatment.—Remove any unabsorbed poison from the **stomach by emetics** or **stomach-pump**. The best *antidote* * is freshly precipitated ferric hydrate, made by adding aqua ammoniæ to a solution of a ferric salt. "Dialysed iron," being a solution of ferric hydrate, may be used. It should be given at frequent intervals and in tablespoonful doses.

TESTS FOR ARSENIC.—*In the solid state:* 1. Heated on a knife-blade over a lamp, it *volatilizes* with a white smoke, and leaves no residue.

2. Heated in a test-tube it *sublimes*, and is recondensed in the cooler portion of the tube (Fig. 24) as *octahedral crystals* (Fig. 25).

3. Heated in a small tube with powdered charcoal, the arsenic is reduced as it sublimes, and recondenses on the cooler portion of the tube in the metallic state.

In the liquid state: 1. Through the solution, acidulated or rendered neutral, pass H_2S; a yellow precipitate (As_2S_3) falls.

---

* An antidote is something harmless and capable of rendering the poison harmless. Since poisons are inert when insoluble, antidotes are usually such substances as are capable of combining with the poison to form an insoluble and therefore inert compound.

2. To an aqueous solution add a few drops of nitrate of silver, and then cautiously add ammonia, drop by drop, till a yellow precipitate, *silver arsenite* (Ag_3AsO_3) is obtained, showing the presence of arsenic.

3. Repeat the preceding, adding copper sulphate instead of silver nitrate, and the presence of arsenic is indicated by a green precipitate of copper arsenite (Scheele's green or Paris green).

The last two tests may be performed with greater ease and delicacy if the silver nitrate and copper sulphate each be previously treated with ammonia until the precipitate first formed is barely dissolved, forming solutions of *ammonio-nitrate of silver* and *ammonio-sulphate of copper*, which are filtered and set aside as test reagents.

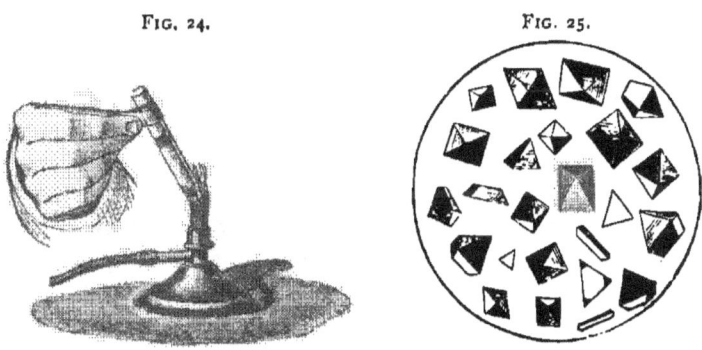

FIG. 24.   FIG. 25.

The Plating (Reinsch's) Test.—Place a thin piece of pure copper in the solution acidulated with HCl, and boil. If arsenic be present, it will be deposited as a metallic film on the copper. If the solution be then poured off, and the piece of copper, carefully dried, be heated in a dry test-tube, the film will sublime and condense on the sides of the tube, and the preceding tests may be applied.

The Hydrogen (Marsh's) Test depends on the fact that AsH_3 is always formed whenever hydrogen is generated in the presence of any arsenical compound. Generate hydrogen (Fig. 26) in the usual way ($Zn + H_2SO_4$), and if the chemicals are pure (free from arsenic), the gas burns with a pale yellowish flame, without odor, and does not stain a porcelain dish held in the flame. Then pour into the generator some of the suspected solution. If arsenic be present, there is an odor of garlic; the flame becomes bluish-white, and a cold porcelain dish held in the jet (Fig. 28) so chills the flame that only the H burns, and the As is deposited on the porcelain as a brilliant metallic film.

FIG. 26.

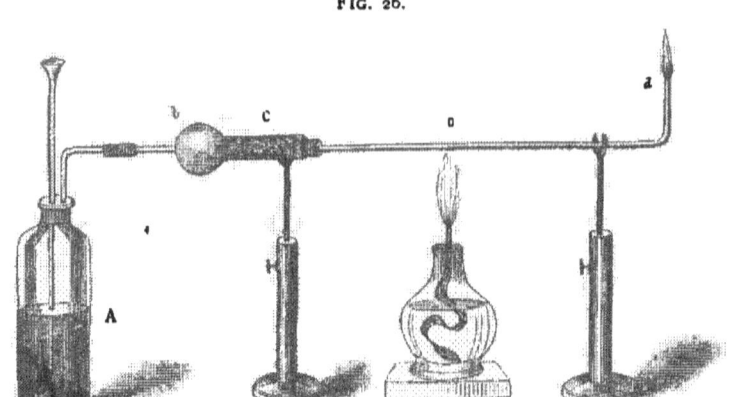

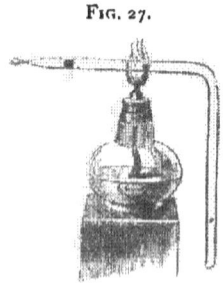

FIG. 27.

If the delivery tube be heated (Fig. 27), the passing AsH$_3$ is decomposed, and metallic arsenic deposits farther out in the tube in a film of the same character as that on the porcelain.

This may be distinguished from the film formed by antimony under similar circumstances by (1) its greater metallic lustre, and (2) by its dissolving on the addition of chlorinated soda (Labarraque's solution); (3) moisten the spot with nitric acid; evaporate the acid; a white stain is left, which is colored a red by AgNO$_3$ and yellow by H$_2$S. The flame should now be extinguished and the delivery-tube made to dip into a solution of AgNO$_3$. This will be blackened, and, if overlaid with aqua ammoniæ, a yellow precipitate will appear at the junction of the two fluids.

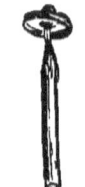

FIG. 28.

ANTIMONY (stibium) *occurs* native, but usually as a sulphide. *Prepared* by roasting the sulphide, and heating the oxide thus obtained with charcoal.

Properties.—A bluish-white, brittle, crystalline solid, with a brilliant metallic lustre. Resembles metals and forms alloys. In chemical properties it plays the *rôle* of positive and negative radical with equal facility.

Used in alloys, as type metal, Babbitt's metal, Britannia, etc., to which it gives hardness and causes them to expand and fill the moulds on solidifying. The metal is not used in medicine, most of the compounds being obtained from the sulphide.

ANTIMONIOUS HYDRIDE.—SbH$_3$ (*Antimoniuretted Hydrogen—Stibine*), corresponding to AsH$_3$.—This gas is formed wherever hydrogen is generated (nascent) in presence of a reducible antimony compound.

ANTIMONIOUS CHLORIDE—SbCl$_3$.—At ordinary temperatures a yellow semi-solid; hence called *butter of antimony*. On addition of considerable water it decomposes, precipitating a white powder, the *oxychloride* (SbO.Cl),* formerly called *powder of algaroth*.

OXIDES AND ACIDS OF ANTIMONY.

$$Sb_2O_3 + H_2O = 2HSbO_2 \text{—(meta) Antimonious acid.}$$
$$Sb_2O_5 + H_2O = 2HSbO_3 \text{—(meta) Antimonic acid.}$$

ANTIMONIOUS OXIDE—Sb$_2$O$_3$.—*Prepared* by treating the oxychloride with sodium carbonate to remove the chlorine. A whitish, insoluble, volatilizable powder.

ANTIMONY AND POTASSIUM TARTRATE—(SbO)K$\overline{T}$† (*Tartar Emetic*). *Prepared* by treating Sb$_2$O$_3$ with the bitartrate of potassium, thus:—

$$2KH\overline{T} + Sb_2O_3 = 2(SbO)K\overline{T} + H_2O.$$

Sweetish, metallic taste; soluble in water and slightly so in alcohol. Dissolved in Sherry wine it forms *vinum antimonii*, U. S. P. It enters also into *unguentum antimonii* and *syrupus scillæ compositus*, U. S. P.

ANTIMONIOUS SULPHIDE—Sb$_2$S$_3$, the principal ore of antimony; *occurs* native in black, lustrous masses. It may be precipitated from any antimonial solution by H$_2$S as an orange powder, which is black when thoroughly dried.

Poisoning by antimony occurs oftenest with tartar emetic, for that salt is used more than all the other compounds of antimony. The

---

* SbO and BiO, called respectively *antimonyl* and *bismuthyl*, are univalent radicals, because two valences of the trivalent element being satisfied by the bivalent O, only one free valence is left.

† ($\overline{T}$) is used to represent the tartaric acidulous radical (C$_4$H$_4$O$_6$).

symptoms are those referable to gastro-enteric irritation. Fortunately the salts of antimony are emetic, and cause spontaneous evacuation of the stomach. Encourage this, and give tannic acid or ferric hydrate, which will form an insoluble compound.

The presence of antimony may be detected by (1) orange precipitate with H_2S; (2) by Marsh's test (see page 52).

BISMUTH *occurs* native and as sulphide. *Prepared* by roasting the sulphide in air, and reducing the resulting oxide with charcoal.

Properties.—A brittle, white metal, with a bronze tint; volatilizes at a white heat. Forms compounds closely analogous to those of Sb, but is more positive, and plays the negative *rôle* with less facility.

Used in alloys; *e.g.*, pewter and stereotyping metal; the latter melts in boiling water.

BISMUTH NITRATE—$Bi3NO_3$.—Formed by treating bismuth with nitric acid. Dissolves in a little water, but if much water be added it decomposes, with precipitation of—

BISMUTH SUBNITRATE—$BiONO_3$ (*Bismuth Oxynitrate*)—a white, tasteless powder, much used in medicine and as a cosmetic (pearl white).

BISMUTH SUBCARBONATE—$(BiO)_2CO_3$.—Similar to the preceding in constitution, properties, and uses.

BISMUTH AND AMMONIUM CITRATE.—Obtained in pearly scales by dissolving the citrate in dilute ammonia-water, evaporating to a syrupy consistence and spreading on glass to dry. Being very soluble it is the preparation used in making the popular elixirs of bismuth.

Physiological.—The bismuth salts are tonic, sedative, mildly astringent and antifermentative. Used to allay gastro-intestinal irritation. Occasionally the irritation is increased from presence of arsenic which unscrupulous manufacturers often fail to remove as the Pharmacopœia directs. When preparations of bismuth are taken, the stools are blackened by the sulphide formed with the H_2S in the intestines. In severe cases of diarrhœa, with acid fermentation, this blackening does not occur, and its reappearance is a sign of improvement.

Tests.—(1) H_2S or NH_4HS gives brownish-black precipitate; (2) the concentrated solution poured into water forms a white precipitate.

V. Carbon Group.

CARBON (*carbo*, a coal),	C,	12
SILICON (*silex*, a flint),	Si,	28
TIN (*Stannum*),	Sn,	118
LEAD (*Plumbum*),	Pb,	207

Each element is bivalent and quadrivalent. The dioxide of each forms with water a dibasic acid:—

$CO_2 + H_2O = H_2CO_3$, Carbonic acid.
$SiO_2 + H_2O = H_2SiO_3$, Silicic acid.
$SnO_2 + H_2O = H_2SnO_3$, Stannic acid.
$PbO_2 + H_2O = H_2PbO_3$, Plumbic acid.

CARBON *occurs free* in its three allotropic forms, diamond, graphite, and coal; *combined* in carbonates and in all animal and vegetable substances. All its forms are probably traceable to organized life.

Diamond.—Geological history unknown; transparent crystalline body of great brilliancy; hardest substance known. Used as a gem and for cutting glass, etc.

Graphite (to write).—Owing to its resemblance to lead it has been called *black lead* or *plumbago;* almost pure carbon. Used for pencils, crucibles, stove polish, etc.

COAL.—*Mineral coal* is a black substance, compact in texture, the remains of vegetable life of past ages. *Charcoal* is obtained by burning heaps of wood with a limited supply of air. The volatile constituents pass off, leaving the carbon as a light, porous substance, retaining the form and structure of the wood. *Animal charcoal* is made by heating animal matters in closed iron retorts. Charcoal, especially animal, is a valuable absorbent of odorous gases* and coloring matters.†

Properties.—Free carbon is solid at all temperatures, and insoluble in all menstrua. Ordinarily, free carbon is unaffected by chemical

---

* Experiment.—Fill a test-tube with ammonia gas over mercury (Fig. 29). Introduce a piece of charcoal recently heated. The gas is absorbed as is shown by the rapid rise of the mercury.

† Experiment.—To a solution of indigo, cochineal, or potassium permanganate or beer in a flask, add some animal charcoal, shake up and filter. The filtrate is colorless, and in case beer is used it has also lost its bitter taste.

agents, but at high temperatures it surpasses all other elements in its avidity for O. Hence it is used to separate the metals from their oxides.*

CARBON MONOXIDE—CO—*occurs* whenever carbon is burned with an insufficient supply of air, as in anthracite stoves and furnaces, and in coal gas, but never occurs in nature.

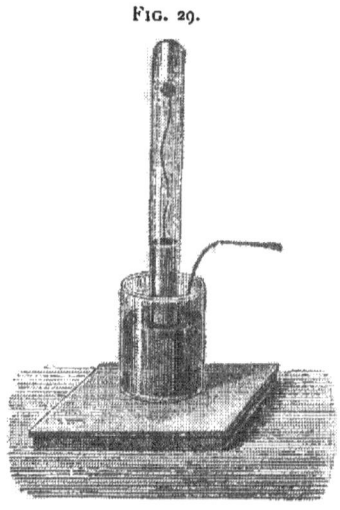

FIG. 29.

Prepared in the laboratory by heating oxalic acid, or potassium ferrocyanide, with sulphuric acid.

Properties. — Colorless, odorless, tasteless gas; burns with a pale blue flame; very poisonous, combining with the coloring matter of the blood corpuscles, and destroying their oxygen-carrying power. Artificial respiration is of little use. Transfusion of blood is the most promising treatment. After death the blood remains scarlet. The sources of danger are open charcoal fires, defective draught in stoves and chimneys, and illuminating gas escaping into bed-rooms.

CARBON DIOXIDE—CO_2.

$$CO_2 + H_2O = H_2CO_3$$—Carbonic acid.

Occurs sparingly (.0004) in the atmosphere, as a result of animal respiration, vegetable decay, and combustion. Plants absorb it, appropriating the carbon and returning the oxygen to the air.

It often accumulates in cellars, beer-vats, wells, etc., where it is called choke-damp.

Prepared by burning carbon, but most conveniently in the laboratory by decomposing a carbonate with an acid.

$$CaCO_3 + 2HCl = CaCl_2 + H_2O + CO_2.$$

Physical Properties.—Transparent, colorless gas, of a pungent odor

---

* **Experiment.**—Into a slight depression in a piece of charcoal lay some metallic oxide—*e. g.*, lead oxide—heat with a blow-pipe. The oxide is reduced by the heated charcoal around it, and globules of the metal appear which coalesce into a bright button.

and sour taste. One and a half times as heavy as air.* Water dissolves its own volume. Soda-water is only a solution of this gas under pressure.†

FIG. 30.

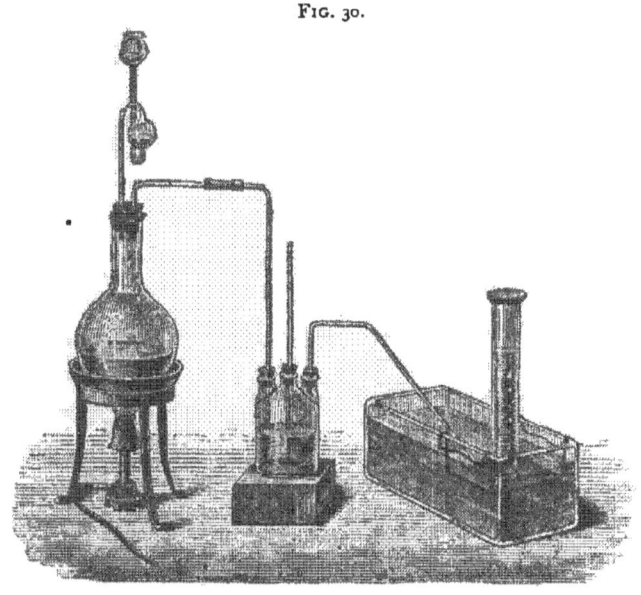

Making CO.

Chemical Properties.—Neither burns nor supports combustion.‡ In water it exists as carbonic acid—H_2CO_3. On attempting to concen-

---

* **Experiments.**—To show the weight of carbon dioxide: (1) Pour it from one vessel to another. (2) Blow soap bubbles and allow them to fall into a wide vessel containing this gas. As soon as they reach the surface of the gas they stop and float upon it. (3) Pour a large beakerful of the gas into a light pasteboard box that has been balanced on a pair of scales. The box will at once descend. This gas accumulating in wells may be bailed in buckets, and tested by being poured upon a lighted candle.

† That water will dissolve a greater quantity of carbon dioxide under pressure is shown by the rapid evolution of the gas whenever a bottle of soda or other carbonated water is opened and the pressure thereby removed.

‡ Set a candlestick, holding several lighted tapers at different heights, in a large jar. Carbon dioxide is introduced at the bottom, and extinguishes the tapers one by one as the vessel fills up to their levels.

trate this dilute solution the acid decomposes again into water and CO_2; hence wet litmus reddened by it becomes blue again on drying.

Tests.—(1) The gas (15 per cent. and over) extinguishes a flame; (2) precipitates lime-water;* (3) carbonates effervesce on adding a strong acid.

Physiological.—If the gas be undiluted, death is immediate from spasm of the glottis. If somewhat dilute (15 to 30 per cent.) there is loss of muscular power, anæsthesia, and death without a struggle. If quite dilute (5 to 10 per cent.) headache, giddiness, muscular weakness, and sometimes vomiting and convulsions occur.

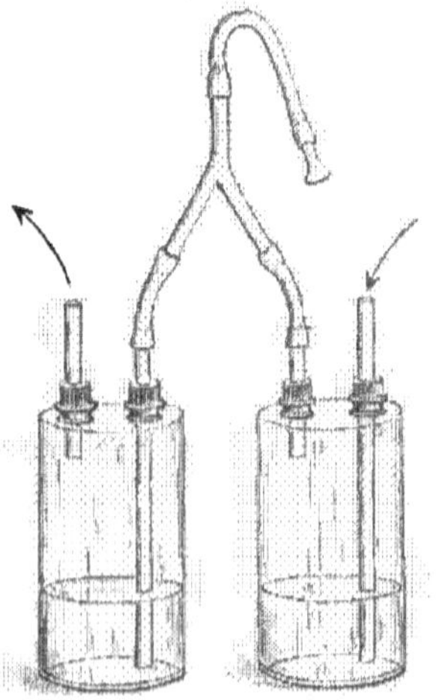

The effects are more serious if the CO_2 comes from combustion or respiration, because of the removal of oxygen and the admixture of the deadly CO and animal exhalations.

Treatment.—Fresh air, artificial respiration, and stimulation. The preventive is ventilation.

FIG. 31.

VENTILATION.—More than 7 parts of CO_2 in 10,000 of air is oppressive. Taking this as the maximum impurity allowable, 3000 cubic feet of fresh air per hour is needed by each person, and more in case of disease or when lamps are burning. To secure this in a room containing 1000 cubic feet ($10 \times 10 \times 10$) the air must be changed three times an hour. This would give a draught not uncomfortable or injurious. If the draught be properly distributed, a breathing space of 500 cubic feet changing six times an hour would be unobjectionable. Ventilation may be secured in two ways, by diffusion and by draught.

---

* Experiment.—Two **Wolff bottles are** half filled with lime-water and arranged as in Fig. 31. Placing the rubber tube in his mouth, the operator can inspire through one bottle and expire through the other. The small amount of carbon dioxide in the inspired and the larger **amount** in the expired air is shown by a white precipitate, slight in **the one and dense** in the other bottle.

60 ESSENTIALS OF CHEMISTRY.

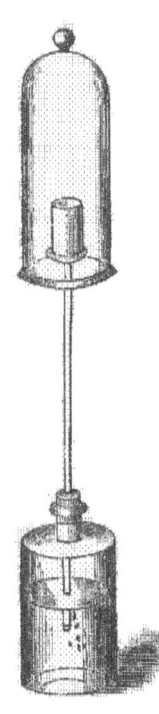

FIG. 32.

Diffusion.—Gases mingle more rapidly, liquids more slowly, to make a mixture of uniform density. When two gases of different densities are separated by a porous partition, they mingle, the lighter passing through more rapidly than the heavier, the rapidity being in inverse ratio to the square roots of their densities.*

This diffusion is more active in winter than in summer, because of the greater difference in density of the warm air within the house and the cold air without. Damp walls are unhealthful mainly because being no longer porous they prevent this diffusion.

CYANOGEN—CN or Cy. Univalent because N^{III} can satisfy only three valences of C^{IV}. A compound negative radical resembling in its chemical behavior the elements of the chlorine group.

Prepared by strongly heating mercuric cyanide.†

$$Hg(CN)_2 = Hg + 2CN.$$

A colorless gas, smelling like peach kernels. Burns with a peach-blossom flame; unites with metals to form cyanides, the most important being—

HYDROCYANIC ACID—H(CN), or HCy—(*Prussic Acid, Hydrogen Cyanide*).—*Occurs* in bitter almonds, cherry-laurel water, etc.

Properties.—Colorless liquid, having an odor like peach kernels.

---

* **Experiment.**—Cement a porous earthenware battery cup at its open end to the top of a funnel tube, the end of which dips into a bottle of colored water. Support on a stand, as in Fig. 32. Bring down over the cup an inverted bell jar of hydrogen. The light H diffuses so much faster into the cup than the air diffuses out of it, that bubbles of gas escape rapidly through the water. Remove the bell jar and the conditions are reversed. The H now diffuses so rapidly out of the cup that the water is sucked up the tube.

† If mercuric cyanide cannot be obtained, a mixture of two parts of thoroughly dried potassium ferrocyanide and three parts mercuric chloride may be used.

PART I.—INORGANIC CHEMISTRY.

For medical purposes only a dilute (2 per cent.) solution is used, and the dose is from two to five drops.

Toxicology.—All the cyanides are very poisonous. One drop of the pure acid produces immediate death, and three grains of potassium cyanide kills in a few minutes. The respiratory centres are paralyzed, and the victim falls and dies in convulsions. Poisoning is liable to occur from handling the acid or the cyanides, which are largely used in the arts, or from eating vegetable products, *e. g.* peach and cherry seeds containing *amygdalin,* a substance easily decomposing into prussic acid and other products. Owing to the rapid action of the poison, antidotes are usually impracticable. Use artificial respiration and stimulate. If the patient survive an hour, the prognosis is good.

Tests.—(1) Its odor; (2) silver nitrate—white precipitate soluble in boiling HNO_3; (3) add ammonium sulphydrate, evaporate to dryness, and then add ferric chloride—a blood-red color.

CYANATES.—Cyanic acid (HCyO) and ammonium cyanate (NH_4-CyO) are the most interesting. The latter on being heated forms urea.

SULPHOCYANATES are sulpho-salts corresponding to the cyanates (oxy-salts), and are good illustrations of the facility with which S forms series of compounds analogous to those of O. They, especially the potassium and sodium salts, are used as test reagents.

COMPOUND CYANIDES.—Cyanogen shows a great tendency to form complex radicals, especially with iron; as, *ferrocyanogen* $[Fe^{II}(CN)_6^{I}]^{IV}$ or $(FeCy_6)^{IV}$, and *ferricyanogen* $[Fe_2^{VI}(CN)_{12}^{I}]^{VI}$ or $(Fe_2Cy_{12})^{VI}$. These two radicals contain ferrous and ferric iron respectively, and with hydrogen form acids known as *hydro-ferrocyanic acid,* H_4FeCy_6 (tetrabasic), and *hydro-ferricyanic acid,* $H_6Fe_2CN_{12}$ or $H_6Fe_2Cy_{12}$ (hexabasic); the salts of these acids are termed ferrocyanides and ferricyanides.

POTASSIUM FERROCYANIDE—K_4FeCy_6—commonly called *yellow prussiate of potash,* and POTASSIUM FERRICYANIDE—K_6FeCy_{12}—*red prussiate of potash,* are important test reagents.

The carbon compounds will be further considered under the head of Organic Chemistry.

SILICON (also called silicium) resembles carbon, and occurs in three allotropic forms corresponding to coal, graphite, and diamond; most abundant element after oxygen. It exists in only a few compounds, but they constitute the larger part of the earth's crust. Its principal compound is—

SILICIC OXIDE—SiO_2—occurring as flint, sand, rock-crystal, etc.; with water it forms silicic acid. Clay, soapstone, asbestos.

Silicates of aluminium and magnesium are very abundant, as clay, soapstone, asbestos, etc. Glass is a mixture of several silicates, usually of sodium, calcium and sometimes lead. It is made by melting sand (SiO_2) with the carbonates or oxides of the metals. The addition of certain metallic oxides gives color; *e. g.*, cobalt gives a blue, manganese an amethyst, and copper a ruby. If the glass consist of only an alkaline silicate (*e. g.*, sodium), it is *soluble* or *water-glass*, which is largely used in surgical dressings.

TIN.—A bluish-white malleable metal,* not corroded by air or water; hence used to form a protective coating for iron and copper. *Tin-ware* is usually sheet-iron coated by being dipped into molten tin. Tin alloyed with lead is easily dissolved, and may cause leadpoisoning.

Tin-foil (thin laminæ of tin) is used in wrapping to exclude air and moisture. Tin enters into the composition of a great many alloys. Powdered tin is sometimes used as an anthelmintic.

---

* THE METALS.—*Occurrence.*—Some, as gold and copper, occur free, but most of them are found combined with non-metallic elements, especially sulphur and oxygen.

Preparation.—If combined with sulphur the ore is roasted until the sulphur is burned out, leaving the metal as an oxide, which is then heated with carbon to remove the oxygen, thus:—

$$ZnS + O_3 = ZnO + SO_2; \text{ then, } ZnO + C = CO + Zn.$$

Physical Properties.—Very opaque, with a "metallic lustre" (in fine powder, a dull black); bluish-gray, varying between the pure white of silver and the dull blue of lead. Yellow gold and red copper are exceptions. In weight, varying between lithium, specific gravity 0.58, and platinum, specific gravity 21.50. Most are solid, except mercury (liquid) and hydrogen (gaseous). All are absolutely insoluble.

Chemical Properties.—Electro-positive, possessing great affinity for the nonmetals and other electro-negative radicals. When two metals are fused together the product is an *alloy*. If one of the metals be mercury, it is called an *amalgam*. Alloys are not chemical compounds, but mixtures, for the metals do not unite in definite proportions, and the alloy is not a new substance, but one with properties intermediate between those of its constituent metals.

Used mostly in the arts. Of the fifty-five metals only about twenty-six, or rather compounds of these, enter the materia medica, and merit our notice.

Tin forms two classes of compounds; the *stannous*, in which the atom is bivalent, and *stannic*, in which the atom is quadrivalent. These are of importance to the chemist, but of little interest to the physician.

LEAD.—Its principal ore is its sulphide (PbS), called *galena*. It is a soft, heavy, blue metal, very slowly acted upon by most substances; hence used to make water-pipes and vessels that are exposed to corrosive liquids.

Water containing nitrates or nitrites (from organic matter) dissolves lead slightly; but if it contains carbonates or sulphates, the lead is protected by an insoluble coating of lead carbonate or sulphate.

Lead enters into the composition of many alloys: as pewter, solder, shot, type-metal, etc. The quadrivalent compounds of lead are of so little importance that the term *plumbic* is applied to the bivalent compounds.

LEAD OXIDE—PbO—*Litharge.*—A yellow substance, found native; made artificially by heating lead in the air. It is by treating this with the appropriate acid that most of the lead salts are prepared. When rubbed with oil it decomposes the glyceryllic ethers and combines with the fatty acids to form lead soaps, one of which, the oleate, is *lead plaster, emplastrum plumbi*, U. S. P.

LEAD DIOXIDE, or *puce lead*, is a dark-brown powder, forming one of the constituents of *red lead* (Pb_3O_4 or $2PbO.PbO_2$).

Prepared by treating *red lead* with nitric acid to dissolve out the PbO.

LEAD NITRATE—$Pb2NO_3$.
Made: $PbO + 2HNO_3 = Pb2NO_3 + H_2O$.

Ledoyen's disinfectant fluid is a solution of $Pb2NO_3$ (one drachm to the ounce). It corrects fetid odors by neutralizing H_2S and NH_4HS.

LEAD ACETATE—$Pb(C_2H_3O_2)_2$, or $PbAc_2$—*Sugar of Lead.*
Made: $PbO + 2HAc = PbAc_2 + H_2O$.

Used in medicine more than any other lead salt. Its solution will dissolve considerable quantities of PbO, forming the *solution of the subacetate of lead, the liquor plumbi subacetatis*, U. S. P., *Goulard's extract*. It is astringent, and, like all the lead salts, sedative. Much used as a topical application in erysipelas, acute eczema, and other skin affections; and diluted (*lead-water*), it is used in conjunctivitis and other mucous inflammations.

The following insoluble salts may be made by precipitation from solutions of the preceding soluble ones:—

LEAD CHLORIDE—$PbCl_2$.—*Made:* Soluble lead salt added to a soluble chloride; *e. g.*, $PbAc_2 + 2HCl = PbCl_2 + 2HAc$. Slightly soluble in warm water, but in cold it is always precipitated from solutions of moderate strength; hence classed with HgCl and AgCl as one of the three insoluble chlorides.

LEAD SULPHATE—$PbSO_4$.—Forms as a white precipitate whenever a solution of a lead salt is added to a sulphate solution, thus:—

$$PbAc_2 + ZnSO_4 = PbSO_4 + ZnAc_2.$$

LEAD CARBONATE—$PbCO_3$—*White Lead.*
Made: $PbAc_2 + Na_2CO_3 = PbCO_3 + 2NaAc$.
Commercially, it is made by some modification of the old Dutch method, which consists in covering bars of lead with the refuse of the wine-press and barn manure. The acetic fumes from the grape husks attack the lead, forming lead acetate, which is decomposed by the carbonic acid from the manure. The acetic acid thus liberated combines with another portion of lead, which is again precipitated by the carbonic acid, and thus the process continues until all the lead is consumed.

Used for painting, but blackens when air contains H_2S.

LEAD SULPHIDE—PbS—is formed as a black precipitate whenever a lead solution is treated with a soluble sulphide, as H_2S or NH_4HS.

LEAD IODIDE—PbI_2.—A bright yellow precipitate on adding a soluble iodide to a lead solution; as,—

$$PbAc_2 + 2KI = 2KAc + PbI_2.$$

LEAD CHROMATE—$PbCrO_4$.
Made: $PbAc_2 + K_2CrO_4 = PbCrO_4 + 2KAc$.
Under the name of *chrome yellow* it is used in painting. Of late it has been used to color food products.

Tests for lead consist in forming precipitates of the foregoing insoluble compounds.

Physiological.—All the lead compounds are poisonous. *Acute* poisoning sometimes occurs from the ingestion of a single large dose of a soluble lead salt. The symptoms are those of gastric irritation. *Treatment.* Give $MgSO_4$ to form the insoluble $PbSO_4$.

The *chronic* form of lead intoxication, *painter's colic*, is purely poisonous, and is produced by the continued absorption of minute quantities of lead by the skin of those handling it, and by the lungs and stomachs of those living in painted apartments, or using food and drink from leaden vessels. There is impairment of digestion, constipation, blue line along the edge of the gums, colic, and paralysis, especially of the extensor muscles. Lead once absorbed is eliminated very slowly, having combined with the albuminoids, a combination which is rendered soluble by the administration of iodide of potassium.

The *treatment* for chronic lead-poisoning is to give $MgSO_4$, for the double purpose of overcoming the constipation and precipitating any lead remaining unabsorbed in the alimentary canal; also KI to promote the elimination of that which is combined with the albuminoids. Alum is a favorite treatment, seeming to perform all accomplished by both the $MgSO_4$ and KI. The paralyzed muscles must be treated with electricity, so that when the lead is eliminated and the nerve influence returns, it may not find them degenerated past redemption.

VI. Metals of the Alkalies.

Hydrogen,	H	1
Lithium,	Li	7
Ammonium,	(NH_4)	18
Sodium (Natrium),	Na	23
Potassium (Kalium),	K	39.1
Rubidium,	Rb	85
Cæsium,	Cs	133.

Univalent; very electro-positive (except H), so that when combined, unless it be with a strongly electro-negative (acidulous) radical, they form very alkaline compounds (hence the name). The positive affinities, as in the other groups, increase with the atomic weights. All their compounds are soluble.

LITHIUM.—Sparingly but widely distributed in nature, especially in the waters of certain springs. Lightest of the solid elements. Its salts closely resemble those of sodium.

Physiological.—Lithium urate being by far the most soluble compound of uric acid, salts of lithium, especially the carbonate, are given to gouty persons to promote the elimination of uric acid, which accumulates in that disease.

Test.—It colors the flame a beautiful carmine red.

AMMONIUM.—When ammonia gas (NH_3) combines with an acid, it appropriates the basic hydrogen and forms a salt in which NH_4 is the positive radical; *e. g.*:—

$NH_3 + HCl = NH_4Cl$, corresponding to KCl or NaCl;
$NH_3 + HHO = NH_4HO$, corresponding to KHO or NaHO;
$NH_3 + HNO_3 = NH_4NO_3$, corresponding to KNO_3 or $NaNO_3$;
$2NH_3 + H_2SO_4 = (NH_4)_2SO_4$, corresponding to K_2SO_4 or Na_2SO_4.

This radical plays the *rôle* of a metal, like K and Na, and is called *Ammonium*. Does not exist uncombined, although Weyl claims to isolate it as a dark-blue liquid metal.* We can obtain it as an amalgam by the reaction between sodium amalgam and ammonium chloride.†

AMMONIUM HYDRATE—NH_4HO—*Caustic Ammonia*—is formed in solution whenever ammonia gas (NH_3) dissolves in water, thus: $NH_3 + H_2O = NH_4HO$. It has been already stated that the watery solution of a fixed substance is called a *liquor;* of a volatile substance, an *aqua*. In like manner alcoholic solutions of fixed substances are called *tinctures*, and of volatile, *spirits*. There are four U. S. P. solutions of ammonia:—

Aqua ammoniæ, ... *10 per cent.*
Aqua ammoniæ fortior, ... 26 "
Spiritus ammoniæ, ... *10* "
Spiritus ammoniæ aromaticus.

---

* Experiment.—*The supposed free ammonium.* Sodio-ammonium is prepared by heating sodium in a sealed tube with ammonia gas. This is in turn heated with ammonium chloride in a sealed tube. A dark blue liquid, with metallic lustre, is obtained, but soon decomposes into ammonia gas and hydrogen.

† Experiment.—To some mercury in a test-tube add sodium, small bits at a time. On this sodium amalgam pour a strong solution of ammonium chloride. Sodium chloride and ammonium amalgam are formed.

$$(Na + Hg) + NH_4Cl = NaCl + (NH_4 + Hg).$$

The ammonium amalgam swells up and soon decomposes—$(NH_4 + Hg) = NH_3 + H + Hg$—the gaseous NH_3 and hydrogen escape, and only the mercury remains.

PART I.—INORGANIC CHEMISTRY. 67

In all these solutions NH_4HO exists, but has never been isolated, because, whenever we attempt to evaporate the water or alcohol, the NH_4HO decomposes into $NH_3 + H_2O$. Ammonium hydrate is very alkaline.

AMMONIUM HYDROSULPHIDE—NH_4HS—*occurs* in decomposing nitrogenous, sulphurized organic bodies. *Made* by saturating a solution of NH_4HO with H_2S. A yellowish solution; used as a test reagent.

AMMONIUM CARBONATE—$(NH_4)_2CO_3$.—*Ammonii Carbonas*, U. S. P. —*Sal volatile*—is prepared by heating a mixture of NH_4Cl and chalk ($CaCO_3$) up to the temperature at which $(NH_4)_2CO_3$ would be volatilized, when the following reaction will occur:—

$$2NH_4Cl + CaCO_3 = CaCl_2 + (NH_4)_2CO_3.$$

(See *Volatility*, page 25.) Very prone to absorb CO_2 from the atmosphere and become bicarbonate unless NH_4HO be added.

OTHER SALTS may be made by adding the appropriate acid to the carbonate or hydrate of ammonium. If we use the carbonate, we can tell when acid enough has been added by the cessation of effervescence. If the hydrate be used there is no effervescence, and our only guide is the point at which the solution becomes neutral in reaction. This is determined by the use of test papers. These are made of white, unsized paper, steeped in a blue vegetable pigment called *litmus*, which is *reddened* by *acids* and *restored* to its *blue* by *alkalies*.

Physiological.—The hydrate and carbonate are alkaline irritants, like the corresponding K and Na compounds, though in less degree. They, moreover, give off NH_3, which, though irritating to the respiratory tract, is a valuable stimulant in fainting fits, etc. Two drachms of aqua ammoniæ have killed. The treatment, as *for all alkalies*, is to give a dilute acid or some oil.

Tests.—(1) An ammonium salt warmed with liq. potassæ gives off NH_3, recognized (*a*) by its odor, (*b*) its forming a white cloud of NH_4Cl when a glass rod dipped in the HCl is held over the vessel, and (*c*) its changing moist red litmus to blue. (2) Heat the dry ammonium salt and it volatilizes.

SODIUM *occurs* very abundantly as sodium chloride, or common salt, from which almost all the sodium compounds are now obtained instead of from ashes of seaweeds, as formerly. The *preparation* and *properties* of sodium and its compounds are so similar to those of potassium that we will omit their separate consideration. So much alike are the salts of the two metals that the choice between them is usually governed by considerations of economy, convenience, solubility, fashion, etc. On exposure to the atmosphere the sodium salts usually have a tendency to *effloresce*, while the potassium salts tend to *deliquesce*.

Tests.—No good precipitant; for all the compounds of sodium are soluble. However, the strong yellow color it gives a flame is a very delicate test; in fact, too delicate, for it shows traces of sodium in almost everything.

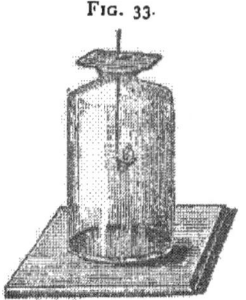

FIG. 33.

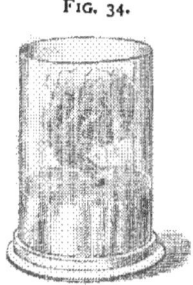

FIG. 34.

POTASSIUM *occurs* only in compounds. *Prepared* by heating one of its oxygen compounds with charcoal in an iron retort ($K_2CO_3 + 2C = 3CO + K_2$). The metallic K distills over and is condensed in a flat receiver.

Physical Properties.—Soft as wax; lighter than water; silvery lustre when freshly cut, but quickly tarnishes.

Chemical Properties.—Intensely electro-positive; hence it possesses great affinity for the non-metals;* takes O from H_2O, even as ice, † setting fire to the escaping H, giving the flame the violet color characteristic of K (Fig. 34).

---

*Experiment.—Potassium inflames spontaneously when lowered into a jar of chlorine (Fig. 33). Warmed with iodine or dropped into bromine it explodes violently. This should be done under a tubulated bell jar, because the potassium is scattered in every direction.

† Experiment.—Load a strong toy cannon with gunpowder. On the fuse lay a small bit of potassium. Touching it with a piece of ice fires the cannon.

POTASSIUM CARBONATE—K_2CO_3.—Obtained as an impure solution ("lye") by lixiviating the ashes of plants, especially forest trees. This, evaporated to dryness, forms "concentrated lye." This in turn, when purified, forms "pearl-ash," which is further purified for medicinal use. Sometimes made by burning cream of tartar and lixiviating the residue, hence called *salts of tartar*. A white semi-crystalline or granular powder. CO_3 being a weakly acidulous radical, K_2CO_3 is very alkaline, even caustic.

ACID SALTS.—Salts are formed by a metallic radical displacing the basic H of an acid. If all the H be displaced, the result is a *normal salt*, as, $H_2SO_4 + K_2 = K_2SO_4 + H_2$. But if part of the basic H of the acid remains, it is called an *acid salt*, as $H_2SO_4 + K = KHSO_4 + H$. Sometimes acid salts are called "bi" salts, because the proportion of the acidulous radical to the basylous is twice as great as in the normal; *e.g.*, $KHSO_4$ is called potassium bisulphate, because the proportion of the acidulous radical SO_4 to the basylous radical K is twice as great as in the normal sulphate, K_2SO_4.

POTASSIUM BICARBONATE—$KHCO_3$.—Although an acid salt in constitution, it is alkaline in reaction, on account of the weakness of its acidulous radical. Made by passing CO_2 into a solution of K_2CO_3. The reaction is as follows:—

$$K_2CO_3 + H_2O + CO_2 = 2KHCO_3.$$

POTASSIUM BITARTRATE—$KH(C_4H_4O_6)$ or $K\overline{HT}$—*Cream of Tartar*.—Prepared similarly to the above, by adding tartaric acid to a solution of the normal tartrate, thus: $K_2\overline{T} + H_2\overline{T} = 2K\overline{HT}$. It exists naturally in grape juice, and, being insoluble in an alcoholic menstruum, is precipitated on the sides of the wine casks whenever vinous fermentation sets in. This is its commercial source.

OTHER SALTS.—Most salts of K are made by treating the carbonate with the appropriate acid, *e.g.*:—

The chloride—$K_2CO_3 + 2HCl = 2KCl + H_2O + CO_2$.
The sulphate—$K_2CO_3 + H_2SO_4 = K_2SO_4 + H_2O + CO_2$, etc.

The decomposition is attended with an effervescence of CO_2. It is the formation of this volatile compound that determines the reaction. (See *Volatility*, page 25.)

But the following salts are not made in this way:—

POTASSIUM HYDRATE—KHO—*Caustic Potash*—may be made experimentally by the reaction of metallic K on water, thus:—

$$H_2O + K = KHO + H.$$

But made in the shops by boiling K_2CO_3 with slaked lime, thus:—

$$K_2CO_3 + Ca2HO = CaCO_3 + 2KHO.$$

The insoluble $CaCO_3$ (chalk) sinks to the bottom, and the KHO dissolves in the supernatant liquid, which when clear is poured off (decanted). This watery solution, if of proper strength (℥j–Oj), forms "*Liquor potassæ*, U. S. P." If this solution be evaporated to a syrupy consistence and poured into moulds, it forms the stick caustic potash. KHO is very alkaline, and a powerful cautery.

Exposed to the air it absorbs CO_2 and forms carbonate:—

$$2KHO + CO_2 = K_2CO_3 + H_2O.$$

POTASSIUM IODIDE—KI:—

$$6KHO + 6I = 5KI + KIO_3 + 3H_2O.$$

The color disappears because the I goes to form colorless salts. Prepared thus, the KI is contaminated with KIO_3 (K-Iodate).* But if the mixture be strongly heated the O_3 is driven off and the KI alone remains. The addition of charcoal facilitates the removal of the O_3.

POTASSIUM BROMIDE—KBr—may be made similarly to the above.

SODIO-POTASSIUM TARTRATE—NaKT—*Rochelle Salt.*—A neutral salt made by boiling acid potassium tartrate with sodium bicarbonate.

$$KHT + NaHCO_3 = NaKT + H_2O + CO_2.$$

This is the reaction that occurs in baking with cream of tartar baking powders.

POTASSIUM HYPOCHLORITE—KClO.—Made by passing chlorine into a cold solution of KHO. Yields free chlorine. The ordinary bleach-

---

* Experiment.—The presence of KIO_3 in a commercial specimen of KI may be recognized by boiling a little starch in a test-tube, dissolving a crystal of the suspected salt, and then adding a few drops of a strong solution of tartaric acid; if KIO_3 be present, I will be liberated, and a blue color struck with the starch.

ing solutions (Labarraque's Solution or Javelle water) are solutions of impure sodium or potassium hypochlorite.

Tests for Potassium.—(1) If the suspected solution be concentrated, add H_2T and get a precipitate of KHT.* (2) Platinic chloride ($PtCl_4$) gives a yellowish precipitate. But the $PtCl_4$ is very costly, and all the potassium compounds so soluble that the above tests are but little used. The most convenient is the (3) flame test : dip the end of a clean platinum wire in the suspected solution, and hold in the colorless Bunsen or alcohol flame and notice the violet color.

CÆSIUM AND RUBIDIUM.—Rare metals, occurring in small quantities with potassium. Discovered in 1860 by means of the spectroscope, and named from the colors of their lines in the spectrum (*cæsius*, sky blue, and *rubidus*, dark red). Of no medical interest as yet.

Analytical.—To determine whether a salt be a compound of K, Na, NH_4, or Li, heat samples of each ; the one that volatilizes is the salt of NH_4. Confirm this by boiling with KHO and getting the odor of ammonia. To the other three salts apply the flame tests, getting the violet for K,† yellow for Na, and carmine for Li.

VII. Metals of the Alkaline Earths.

MAGNESIUM,	Mg	24
CALCIUM,	Ca	40
STRONTIUM,	Sr	87.5
BARIUM,	Ba	137

Bivalent; their oxides and hydrates are very *alkaline*, but of an *earthy* character. Their positiveness or basicity, as in other groups, is in the order of the atomic weights. Their carbonates are decomposable by heat and insoluble in water, unless it contains H_2CO_3 in solution. Their sulphates increase in solubility from the insoluble barium salt to the very soluble magnesium sulphate.

MAGNESIUM.—Never free ; abundant in magnesian limestone ($CaCO_3.MgCO_3$). Asbestos, meerschaum, and soapstone are native

---

* The addition of alcohol renders the test much more delicate.

† The delicate violet of K may be masked by the intense yellow of Na, but can be seen if observed through a piece of blue glass, a medium that absorbs the yellow light.

silicates. Most natural waters contain its salts. Silvery white metal; burns with a brilliant white light, rich in chemical rays, and used in photographing caves and other dark places.

MAGNESIUM SULPHATE—$MgSO_4$—*occurs* in the waters of various springs, as those at Epsom; hence often called *Epsom salts*. Made artificially from the native carbonate, thus:—

$$MgCO_3 + H_2SO_4 = MgSO_4 + (H_2O + CO_2).$$

White, crystalline, soluble salt of a nauseous bitter taste. It is a popular purgative. The nauseous taste and griping may be obviated by adding aromatics, acid, sulphate of iron (as in Crab Orchard salts), or by free dilution.

MAGNESIUM CITRATE is the most pleasant of the saline purgatives. Usually given as the *liquor magnesii citratis*, which is prepared by adding a solution of citric acid to $MgCO_3$, and bottling immediately to retain the CO_2.

MAGNESIUM CARBONATE—$MgCO_3$—*occurs* native. For medicinal purposes it is prepared by precipitation, thus:—

$$MgSO_4 + Na_2CO_3 = Na_2SO_4 + MgCO_3.$$

Similar to chalk in its physical and chemical properties.

MAGNESIUM OXIDE—MgO—*Magnesia*. Made like CaO, by heating the carbonate.

$$MgCO_3 = MgO + CO_2.$$

Insoluble and tasteless (earthy), but its alkalinity is shown by its turning moist red litmus paper blue when the solid MgO is dropped upon it.

MAGNESIUM HYDRATE — $Mg(HO)_2$. — Formed by precipitating a magnesium solution with potassium or sodium hydrate. Insoluble in water, but, like other salts of magnesium, soluble in the presence of ammonium compounds with which they form double salts. Suspended in water, it is called *milk of magnesia*.

MAGNESIUM PHOSPHATES.—These resemble the calcium phosphates and are associated with them in the body, though in small quantity. The *ammonio-magnesium phosphate* ($MgNH_4PO_4$) is precipitated whenever a soluble phosphate in neutral or alkaline solution finds itself in presence of an ammonium salt, as occurs in the alkaline fermentation of urine.

PART I.—INORGANIC CHEMISTRY. 73

Physiological.—Magnesium oxide and hydrate being alkaline and tasteless, are popular antidotes for acids. These and the carbonate are given to correct acid conditions of the digestive tract, and combining with the acids they form soluble salts that are laxative.

CALCIUM.—Never free, but its compounds are very abundant, as limestone, gypsum, etc. Calcium salts are necessary to animal life, the teeth and bones consisting mainly of calcium phosphate.

CALCIUM CHLORIDE—$CaCl_2$.
Made: $CaCO_3 + 2HCl = CaCl_2 + H_2O + CO_2$.
A white salt; very avid of water and deliquescent; used to dry gases.

CALCIUM CARBONATE—$CaCO_3$.—Abundant as limestone, marble, corals, chalk, and shells of the crustacea, mollusks, etc. Chalk consists of microscopic shells. *Precipitated chalk* is made by adding a soluble carbonate to a soluble calcium salt, as:—

$$Na_2CO_3 + CaCl_2 = 2NaCl + CaCO_3.$$

The precipitate ($CaCO_3$) may be separated from the $CaCl_2$ in solution, by—

(*a*) *Filtration.*—Pouring the mixture into a cone of filter paper placed in a funnel, when the water with the dissolved salt will pass through, leaving the insoluble portion (the precipitate) on the filter. (*b*) *Decantation.*—Allowing the precipitate to settle to the bottom, and pouring off the clear fluid. In either case the precipitate may be washed from any remaining $CaCl_2$ by adding pure water and repeating the process.

CALCIUM OXIDE—CaO—*Lime, quicklime; calx*, U. S. P.—A white solid; made by heating limestone in rude furnaces called kilns.

$$CaCO_3 = CaO + CO_2.$$

When water is added to CaO there is a violent chemical union, great heat is evolved, and a hydrate is formed, thus:—

$$CaO + H_2O = Ca2HO.$$

CALCIUM HYDRATE—Ca2HO—*Slaked lime.*—A white, odorless powder; very slightly soluble in water, less than one grain to the ounce, but enough to give "lime-water" (*liquor calcis*, U. S. P.) a decidedly alkaline taste and reaction. The presence of sugar greatly increases its solubility (*liq. calcis saccharatus*, Br.).

CHLORINATED LIME — *Chloride of lime, bleaching powder*, *calx chlorata*, U. S. P.—is a mixture of chloride of calcium ($CaCl_2$) and calcium hypochlorite (Ca2ClO). It is made by passing chlorine gas over slaked lime until it ceases to be absorbed. It is white, moistens on exposure to the air, absorbing CO_2 and giving off Cl. It is employed as a source from which to get a gradual supply of chlorine for disinfecting and bleaching purposes.

CALCIUM SULPHATE—$CaSO_4$—*occurs* negative, as gypsum, which, when heated, loses its water of crystallization and forms a white amorphous powder called *plaster-of-Paris*. If this plaster be mixed with water enough to form a creamy liquid, it will recrystallize or "set" into a hard compact mass. Much used in surgery to make casts to hold broken limbs in position. Very slightly soluble in water.

CALCIUM PHOSPHATE—$Ca_3(PO_4)_2$.—It is the most abundant mineral ingredient of the body; in every tissue and fluid, especially the teeth and bones, to which it gives hardness and rigidity. A white tasteless powder, soluble in dilute acids. Dissolved by lactic acid, it is given as *syrupus calcii lactophosphatis*, U. S. P., in scrofula, rickets, and other diseases of defective nutrition.

CALCIUM OXALATE—CaC_2O_4, or $CaO\bar{x}$—*occurs* in the juices of some plants and in the urine. Obtained as a fine white crystalline powder when a soluble oxalate is added to a calcium solution. Insoluble in water or acetic acid, but soluble in the mineral acids.

HARD WATERS are such as contain mineral matters, especially calcium (lime) compounds. Often water, in passing through the soil, becomes highly charged with carbonic acid, and dissolves considerable amounts of $CaCO_3$, and is hard. This is called *temporary hardness*, because on exposure or boiling, the carbonic acid is driven off, the $CaCO_3$ is precipitated, and the water becomes *soft*. The solubility of $CaSO_4$ does not depend on the presence of carbonic acid, and boiling will not precipitate it. So water impregnated with $CaSO_4$ is said to be *permanently hard*. Drinking-water should contain a small quantity of lime; but very hard water impairs digestion. Hard water is unfit for washing, because the soluble alkali soap reacts with the lime salt to form an insoluble lime-soap.

PART I.—INORGANIC CHEMISTRY. 75

STRONTIUM.—Of little importance, except that its nitrate is used in pyrotechny to make the red light.*

BARIUM.—Of little interest to the medical student, except that its compounds are poisonous. Barium sulphate is very insoluble; hence (1) the antidote of barium is some soluble sulphate, and (2) barium solutions (nitrate and chloride) are delicate tests for sulphates, and *vice versâ*. (See *Insolubility*, page 26.) Barium gives the flame a green color; hence used (nitrate) in pyrotechny to make the green or Bengal light.†

Analytical.—To determine whether a solution be one of barium, calcium or magnesium: Add potassium chromate; a precipitate indicates *barium*. If no precipitate, add ammonium chloride and then ammonium carbonate; a precipitate indicates *calcium*. If no precipitate, add sodium phosphate; a precipitate indicates *magnesium*.

VIII. Metals of the Earths.

BORON,	B	11
ALUMINIUM,	Al	27
Scandium,	Sc	44
Yttrium,	Y	92
Lanthanum,	La	139
CERIUM,	Ce	141
Didymium,	D	145
Samarium,	Sm	150
Erbium,	E	168
Ytterbium,	Yb	173

Trivalent, though in compounds two atoms go together, forming a

---

* *Red Fire:* Strontium nitrate, 800 grains; sulphur, 225 grains; potassium chlorate, 200 grains, and lampblack, 50 grains.

† *Green Fire:* Barium nitrate, 450 grains; sulphur, 150 grains; potassium chlorate, 100 grains, and lampblack, 25 grains.

For lecture-room experiments the following, without sulphur, are preferable:
Green Fire: Two parts barium nitrate, two parts potassium chlorate, and one part ground shellac.
Red Fire: Two parts strontium nitrate, two parts potassium chlorate, and one part ground shellac.
The ingredients should be *dry*, powdered separately, and mixed with as little friction as possible.

sexivalent radical, as Al_2Cl_6. Boron is so weakly positive that it is a non-metal. Aluminium is the most important member of this group, the others being rare metals associated with it in various minerals. Their oxides and hydrates are of a neutral or earthy character.

BORON *occurs* as a constituent of boracic acid and borax (sodium borate, U. S. P.). Has two allotropic forms, amorphous and crystalline, corresponding to coal and diamond. Forms only one oxide (B_2O_3), which, combining with water, forms an acid:—

$$B_2O_3 + 3H_2O = H_6B_2O_6 = 2H_3BO_3\text{—Boric acid.}$$

BORIC OR BORACIC ACID *occurs* as pearly scales, soluble in water; feebly acid; an unirritating antiseptic. Boiled with glycerine it was sold as *boroglyceride*, or mixed with borax as *rex magnus* to preserve foods, especially milk and meats.

Test.—Compounds of boron, especially when moistened with sulphuric acid, color the flame green.

ALUMINIUM.—Never found free, but in the abundance and distribution of its compounds it ranks next to oxygen and silicon—third among the elements and first among the metals. Isolated with difficulty, and therefore costly. Bluish-white metal, ductile and very light; does not tarnish in the air. With copper it forms a golden-yellow alloy, known as *aluminium bronze*.

ALUMINIUM CHLORIDE—Al_2Cl_6.—*Prepared* industrially in the manufacture of aluminium. A soluble, astringent salt. It absorbs and combines with H_2S, PH_3, and NH_3. An impure solution is sold as a disinfectant under the name *chloralum*.

ALUMINIUM SULPHATE—Al_23SO_4.—Made by treating white clay with H_2SO_4. It has properties similar to the above.

ALUM—*Alumen.*—An alum is a double sulphate of a trivalent and a univalent radical. Its constitution may be expressed thus:—

$$R_2{}^{III}3SO_4.R_2{}^{I}SO_4, \text{ or } 2R^{III}R^I2SO_4.$$

The trivalent radical (R^{III}) may be Al, Fe, Cr, or Mn. The univalent radical (R^I) may be K, Na, NH_4, etc. So, by different combinations of these radicals a variety of alums may be formed. The old *potash alum* ($Al_23SO_4.K_2SO_4$) is giving place in the arts to the cheaper *ammonium alum* ($Al_23SO_4.(NH_4)_2SO_4$). The *ammonio-ferric alum* ($Fe_2 3SO_4.(NH_4)_2SO_4$) is also much used in medicine. Burnt alum, *alumen exsiccatum*, is a white amorphous powder obtained by heating alum until its water of crystallization is driven off. Alum, like other salts in which the acidulous radical predominates, is astringent; burnt alum, on account of its avidity for water, is a mild escharotic.

ALUMINIUM SILICATES.—Very abundant, as granite, clay, sand, etc. Clay is usually of a reddish or brown color from admixture of oxides of Fe, etc. Pure white clay (*kaolin*) is used in the arts to make porcelain, and in medicine as a vehicle for the external application of acids, etc.

CERIUM is a rare metal. One of its salts, the oxalate, is used as a sedative to irritable stomachs, especially in the vomiting of pregnancy. When pure it is a very efficient remedy; but the commercial article is liable to contain salts of lanthanum, didymium, and other allied metals.

The other members of this group possess little interest for the medical student.

IX. The Zinc Group.

ZINC, ... Zn 65.2
CADMIUM, ... Cd 112

Bivalent; bluish-white metals, closely allied in sources and properties.

ZINC.—When heated in air, zinc burns with an intense bluish-white light, forming clouds of oxide. It tarnishes quickly in air or water, but becomes coated with a film of oxide that protects it from further corrosion. Iron coated with zinc ("galvanized iron") will withstand exposure to the weather an indefinite time. Alloyed with copper, zinc forms brass. Pure H_2SO_4 is unaffected by pure zinc or zinc coated with mercury (amalgamated), unless it form a galvanic circuit.* Commercial zinc is rapidly attacked by most acids.

---

* Experiment.—Into a large test-tube containing bits of zinc pour dilute sulphuric acid; there is a prompt effervescence of hydrogen. Add a little mercury, and agitate; the action ceases. Drop in a piece of copper; it begins again.

ZINC SULPHATE—$ZnSO_4$—*White Vitriol*—is made thus:—

$$Zn + H_2SO_4 = ZnSO_4 + H_2.$$

White, soluble salt, resembling $MgSO_4$ in appearance; astringent and emetic.

ZINC CHLORIDE—$ZnCl_2$.—*Made:* $Zn + 2HCl = ZnCl_2 + H_2$. A white deliquescent salt; strongly astringent; severe caustic. Used as an injection to preserve anatomical subjects.

Each of the following mixtures forms a hard, white mass, used for filling teeth:—

(*a*) A strong solution of zinc chloride with zinc oxide.
(*b*) A strong solution of magnesium chloride with magnesium oxide.
(*c*) Zinc oxide with phosphoric acid (zinc phosphate).

ZINC CARBONATE—$ZnCO_3$—is a white, insoluble powder made by precipitation:—

$$ZnSO_4 + Na_2CO_3 = Na_2SO_4 + ZnCO_3.$$

Used in the arts (*zinc white*) in place of lead carbonate, for it is not blackened by H_2S; in medicine as a dusting powder for excoriated surfaces, and in ointment.

ZINC OXIDE—ZnO—is prepared either by burning metallic zinc* or heating the carbonate, $ZnCO_3 = ZnO + CO_2$.

It is a yellowish-white powder, used *externally* in ointment, *internally* as a tonic and astringent, especially in the night-sweats of phthisis and diarrhœa of children.

ZINC SULPHIDE—ZnS—is precipitated whenever a solution of a zinc salt is added to the solution of a soluble sulphide, unless the solution be acid in reaction. It is the only white sulphide, therefore a test for zinc.

Poisoning.—All the salts of zinc that are soluble in the digestive fluids act as irritant poisons. Sodium chloride and organic acids dissolve metallic zinc, therefore food kept in galvanized iron vessels is more or less poisonous, especially since commercial zinc usually con-

---

* **Experiment.**—Place bits of zinc in a hessian crucible and heat strongly over a triple burner. The metal is volatilized, and the vapor igniting burns with an intense bluish-white flame, yielding white flakes of zinc oxide, the *lana philosophica* (philosopher's wool) of the older chemists.

tains traces of arsenic. For this reason articles intended for toxicological analysis should never be kept in jars with zinc caps.

CADMIUM resembles zinc in its properties and uses, except that its sulphide is yellow and insoluble in acid solutions.

X. The Iron Group.

CHROMIUM,	Cr	52.2
MANGANESE,	Mn	55.0
IRON,	Fe	56.0
COBALT,	Co	58.8
NICKEL,	Ni	58.8

These are hard metals and all more or less magnetic.

By a variation in valence they form two classes of compounds: One in which the atom is *bivalent*, as in ferrous chloride ($FeCl_2$); the other in which the atom is *trivalent*, as in ferric chloride (Fe_2Cl_6). With oxygen they form acidulous radicals, which form the chromates, manganates, and ferrates, with the stronger bases.

CHROMIUM.—So named because all its compounds are colored. The metal is of but little use. Its compounds are of great importance to the chemist and of considerable utility in the arts, but few are used in medicine.

CHROMIUM TRIOXIDE—CrO_3—is made by treating a strong solution of potassium bichromate with sulphuric acid, thus:—

$$K_2Cr_2O_7 + H_2SO_4 = K_2SO_4 + H_2CrO_4 + CrO_3.$$

The CrO_3 separates in crimson prisms. It is a powerful oxidant and a caustic. Sometimes improperly called chromic acid.

CHROMATES.—The principal ones are potassium chromate, K_2CrO_4, a valuable test reagent, and lead chromate, $PbCrO_4$, a yellow pigment.

BICHROMATES are not regular acid or bi-salts, but compounds of a chromate and chromium trioxide. The most important of these is potassium bichromate, $K_2Cr_2O_7$, or $K_2CrO_4.CrO_3$. It forms large, red, soluble crystals. It is added to the sulphuric acid in batteries to oxidize* the nascent hydrogen.

Chromates may be recognized by their color and by the yellow precipitate on the addition of lead acetate.

MANGANESE resembles iron in its properties. Used to alloy iron in the preparation of certain kinds of steel. Its most abundant ore is the

MANGANESE DIOXIDE—MnO_2—*Black Oxide of Manganese*—an insoluble steel-gray powder that readily gives up its extra atom of O. Used in large quantities in the preparation of chlorine and oxygen gas.

MANGANOUS SULPHATE—$MnSO_4$.

$$MnO_2 + H_2SO_4 = MnSO_4 + H_2O + O.$$

A soluble, rose-colored salt.

MANGANOUS SULPHIDE—MnS—is precipitated whenever a solution of a salt of manganese is treated with NH_4HS. It is the only flesh-colored sulphide, hence its formation is a *test* of manganese.

MANGANATES.—If a mixture of KHO, $KClO_3$, and MnO_2 be heated together, there results a green mass of *potassium manganate*, K_2MnO_4. If this be dissolved in distilled water, it forms a green solution, which, on boiling, or even standing awhile, is changed to a purple, due to the formation of *potassium permanganate*, $K_2Mn_2O_8$.

The permanganate † gives up its oxygen so readily to organic matter,

---

* **Experiments.**—The oxidizing action of the chromic salts can be shown in a number of reactions. (*a*) Any organic substance, as sugar, oxalic acid, or a chip of wood, boiled in the sulphuric acid and bichromate mixture, is oxidized, disappearing completely, with evolution of carbon dioxide. (*b*) Rinse out a beaker with strong alcohol, and then drop in a few crystals of chromic acid. The thin layer of alcohol is ignited with the odor of aldehyde. (*c*) Pour a few drops of absolute alcohol on the wick of a spirit lamp, and lay on several crystals of chromic acid. **It ignites.**

† **Experiment.**—Powdered potassium permanganate treated with sulphuric acid gives off ozone. (See page 19.) So powerful an oxidizer is this mixture that alcohol, ether, benzol, carbon disulphide, flowers of sulphur, tannin, etc., are ignited on contact with it.

PART I.—INORGANIC CHEMISTRY. 81

at the same time losing its purple color, that it is used as a test for organic impurity in water and as a disinfectant.

Physiological.—Associated with iron (1 to 20), manganese is a normal constituent of the blood corpuscles; hence its preparations, like those of iron, are blood tonics. Valuable in amenorrhœa.

IRON *occurs* abundantly as oxide, carbonate, and sulphide; occasionally free.

Preparation.—The carbonate or sulphide is first roasted until con-

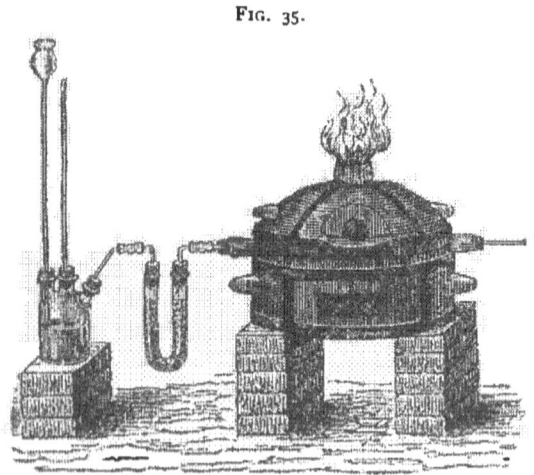

FIG. 35.

Making Reduced Iron.

verted into oxide. The oxide is heated in a blast furnace with coal and fluxes (limestone and silicates). The carbon of the coal removes the oxygen from the iron, which melts and sinks beneath the melted fluxes. The fused metal is then drawn off into furrows in the sand called *pigs*. This is *cast iron*, containing 4 or 5 per cent. of carbon. *Wrought iron* contains little or no carbon, and *steel* an intermediate amount.

Properties.—A bluish-gray metal, sp. gr. 7.5; rusts (oxidizes) when exposed to moist air, or water containing air.

REDUCED IRON—*Ferrum Redactum, iron by hydrogen,* Quevenne's iron.—It is prepared by heating ferric oxide nearly to redness in a tube through which hydrogen is passed:—

$$Fe_2O_3 + H_6 = Fe_2 + 3H_2O.*$$

It is a very fine, dark gray powder, which, if good and fresh, will ignite on contact with a lighted taper and burn with a red glow ; † prescribed in pill form.

CHLORIDES.

FERROUS CHLORIDE—$FeCl_2$.—Made by adding iron to hydrochloric acid until effervescence ceases, thus:—

$$Fe + 2HCl = FeCl_2 + H_2.$$

Like most ferrous salts, it is green and prone to oxidize with the formation of ferric compounds.

FERRIC CHLORIDE—Fe_2Cl_6—is made by first forming the ferrous chloride as above, and then adding nitric and hydrochloric acids. The nascent chlorine evolved by the nitro-hydrochloric acid converts the ferrous into ferric chloride, thus:—

$$6FeCl_2 + 6HCl + 2HNO_3 = 3Fe_2Cl_6 + N_2O_2 + 4H_2O.$$

The *liq. ferri chloridi*, U. S. P., is the aqueous solution. This, when diluted with alcohol, forms the *tinct. ferri chloridi*, U. S. P. If citrate of potassium or sodium be added to this tincture, the solution loses its styptic taste, does not affect the teeth, and is not incompatible with solutions containing tannin.

SULPHATES.

FERROUS SULPHATE—$FeSO_4$.—*Copperas, Green Vitriol.*—Prepared:

---

* **Experiment.**—With the apparatus shown in Fig. 35, hydrogen is generated from sulphuric acid and zinc in the Wolff bottle, and dried by passing through the U-shaped tube containing calcium chloride. It then passes through the porcelain tube containing ferric oxide (subcarbonate, U. S. P.) and is heated to redness in the furnace. After the reduction is completed, the iron should not be exposed to the air until cool, or it will ignite spontaneously.

† **Experiment.**—Faraday used to show that it is more inflammable than gunpowder, by pouring it mixed with gunpowder upon an alcohol flame burning on a white dinner-plate. The iron burns with bright scintillations, while the gunpowder falls through the flame and is only ignited when the flame dies down and reaches the surface of the plate. One part of sulphur, two of reduced iron, and three of nitre make an iron gunpowder that burns as quickly and more brilliantly than ordinary gunpowder.

Fe + H_2SO_4 = $FeSO_4$ + H_2. Soluble, green crystals efflorescing upon exposure. A cheap and excellent disinfectant, destroying organic matters by abstracting their oxygen. When given in pill form it is first *exsiccated*.

FERRIC SULPHATE—Fe_23SO_4.—*Tersulphate* is made by adding nitrosulphuric acid (HNO_3 + H_2SO_4) to a solution of the ferrous sulphate, thus :—

$6FeSO_4 + 3H_2SO_4 + 2HNO_3 = 3Fe_23SO_4 + N_2O_2 + 4H_2O$.

Its officinal solution is the *liq. ferri tersulphatis*. *Liq. ferri subsulphatis*, U. S. P., Monsel's Solution, is prepared similarly to the above, using only half the quantity of sulphuric acid.

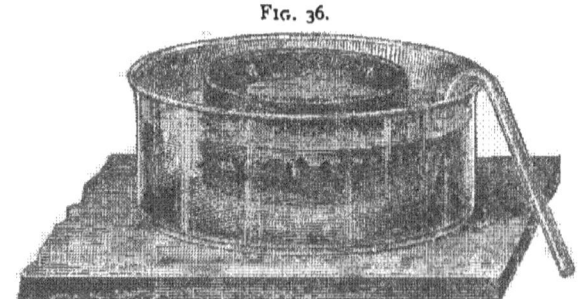

FIG. 36.

A Dialyser.

HYDRATES.

FERROUS HYDRATE—Fe2HO—is precipitated on mixing solutions of a hydrate and a ferrous salt, as—

$FeSO_4 + 2NaHO = Na_2SO_4 + Fe2HO$.

A green precipitate, which soon oxidizes and becomes brown.

FERRIC HYDRATE—Fe_26HO.—A brownish-red, gelatinous mass, precipitated by soluble hydrates from ferric solutions, *e.g.* :—

$Fe_2Cl_6 + 6NH_4HO = 6NH_4Cl + Fe_26HO$.

This is the favorite antidote for arsenic, for which purpose it must be freshly prepared and given in large doses. Ferric hydrate dissolves freely in a solution of ferric chloride, forming a dark red liquid of a styptic taste.

If this liquid be put in a *dialyser* (Fig. 36), a vessel with a bottom of parchment or animal membrane, and suspended in water, the chloride passes out through the membrane into the water. When barely enough ferric chloride remains within the dialyser to hold the ferric hydrate in solution and the styptic taste has disappeared, the liquid is removed and sold under the name of "Dialysed Iron."

FERRIC NITRATE—Fe_26NO_3.
Made: $Fe_26HO + 6HNO_3 = 6H_2O + Fe_26NO_3$.
Liq. ferri nitratis, U. S. P., is a reddish acid liquid. Used as an astringent, especially in dysentery.

FERROUS IODIDE—FeI_2.—Prepared: $Fe + I_2 = FeI_2$.
Sometimes given in pill, but better with syrup, which acts as a preservative as well as a vehicle.

FERROUS CARBONATE—$FeCO_3$—is obtained by adding a soluble (alkaline) carbonate to a ferrous salt, thus:—

$$FeSO_4 + K_2CO_3 = K_2SO_4 + FeCO_3.$$

It is insoluble in pure water, but slightly soluble in water containing carbonic acid, as in chalybeate springs. On exposure to the air it turns red from formation of ferric hydrate; so it is preserved by mixing with sugar and honey, as in the *ferri carbonas saccharatus*, U. S. P.

FERROUS SULPHIDE—FeS—*occurs* native, but may be made by heating together iron filings and flowers of sulphur. Used in the preparation of H_2S.

SCALE COMPOUNDS OF IRON.—These are ferric salts, mostly with organic acids. They do not crystallize readily, but are sold as thin scales. Made by evaporating their solutions to a syrupy consistence, poured upon plates, and when dry peeled off in scales. Often other bases, as potassium or ammonium, together with alkaloids, as quinine and strychnine, are incorporated in the compound.

The following are officinal: *Ferri citras, ferri et ammonii citras, ferri et quiniæ citras, ferri et strychniæ citras, ferri et ammonii tartras, ferri et potassii tartras,* and *ferri pyrophosphas.*

Physiological.—Iron is a normal constituent of the body, especially the blood corpuscles, where it performs an important function, as is shown by the great increase of blood corpuscles and of bodily vigor attending its administration. Many of its salts, especially the ferric salts of the mineral acids, are astringent and hemostatic. Iron is eliminated by various organs, but is mainly discharged by the bowels as sulphide blackening the fæces.

Tests for Iron.—*Ferrous salts* are usually *green ;* with NH_4HS they give a black precipitate of FeS.

Ferric Salts are usually *red;* they give a black precipitate with NH_4HS; a black precipitate with tannic acid; and a blood-red with sulphocyanate of potassium.

COBALT.—Its chief ore is a compound with arsenic, sold under the name of *cobalt* or *flystone,* for poisoning flies. Its salts are used in preparing sympathetic ink, for when free from moisture they are deep blue, but almost colorless when moist. Writing done with a dilute solution of chloride of cobalt is invisible until warmed, when it becomes blue, the color disappearing when the paper is cooled or moistened.

Test for Cobalt.—It imparts a deep blue color to a bead of glass or borax melted in the blow-pipe flame.

NICKEL.—This is a hard, grayish-white metal that does not tarnish in the air. Used to electro-plate instruments made of metals more prone to corrode, and to make cheap coin. Mixed with brass, it forms German silver.

XI. The Copper Group.

COPPER (*Cuprum*), ... Cu 63.4
MERCURY (*Hydrargyrum*), . . Hg 200

Each of these elements is univalent and bivalent, forming two classes of compounds, "*ous*" and "*ic.*" At ordinary temperatures they are acted upon but slowly by the non-oxidizing acids, as H_2SO_4 and HCl; but HNO_3 attacks them vigorously.

COPPER is usually found combined with sulphur, etc., but often in the metallic state, especially on the southern shores of Lake Superior. Being found free, it was among the first metals wrought by man, so the bronze preceded the iron age. Copper is a red malleable metal; an excellent conductor of electricity.

CUPRIC SULPHATE—$CuSO_4$—*Blue Vitriol, Blue Stone.*—Obtained as an incidental product from silver refineries, copper mines, etc.; made experimentally by heating copper with strong H_2SO_4. Forms beautiful blue crystals, soluble in water, but insoluble in alcohol. If the crystals be heated they lose their water of crystallization and form a white powder, which becomes blue again upon the addition of water. Hence, used as a test for water in alcohol. Like other salts in which the acidulous radical predominates, cupric sulphate is astringent and coagulates albumen. A prompt emetic, but not used as much as $ZnSO_4$, because if, by chance, it be not all ejected from the stomach, a gastro-enteritis is liable to be set up.

CUPRIC HYDRATE—Cu2HO—is formed as a bluish-white precipitate whenever a soluble copper salt is treated with a soluble hydrate, thus:

$$CuSO_4 + 2KHO = K_2SO_4 + Cu2HO.$$

When heated, even under water, it decomposes—

$$Cu2HO = CuO + H_2O.$$

CUPRIC OXIDE—CuO—*Black Oxide.*—*Prepared* by heating copper turnings in air. It gives up its oxygen easily, hence used as an oxidizer in organic analysis.

CUPROUS OXIDE—Cu_2O—*Suboxide.*—*Made* by boiling the cupric oxide with an oxidizable substance, as glucose (copper tests for glucose), which is oxidized at the expense of the oxygen of the cupric oxide. The precipitate is first yellow (hydrate), but soon becomes a bright red (oxide).

CUPRIC SUBACETATE OR OXYACETATE—sometimes called *verdigris* (green-gray)—is made industrially by exposing plates of copper to the acetic fumes of grape husks, etc. It is apt to be formed whenever fruits containing acetic acid are placed in copper vessels.

TESTS.—1. *Plating Test.* Dip into the suspected solution a more electro-positive metal, as iron, and a plating of metallic copper will be deposited on the iron, an equivalent proportion of which takes the place of the copper in the solution.

2. *Sulphur Test.* Add H_2S or NH_4HS, and if copper be present a black precipitate (CuS) will be formed.

3. *Ammonia Test.* Add ammonia, and if copper be present a deep blue ammonio-salt of copper will be formed.

4. *Arsenic Test.* To the ammonio-salt, described above, add an aqueous solution of As_2O_3, and a green precipitate of *arsenite of copper* (Paris green) will be thrown down.

5. *Glucose Test.* Add KHO, ($CuSO_4 + 2KHO = K_2SO_4 + Cu2HO$) and boil ($Cu2HO = CuO + H_2O$), with a little glucose, and a yellowish-red precipitate (Cu_2O) indicates copper.

It will be seen from the last two reactions, above described, that a substance acted upon characteristically by a reagent is as good a test for the reagent as the reagent is for it—*i. e.*, arsenic and glucose, being acted upon characteristically by copper, are as good tests for copper as copper is for them.

Physiological.—Canned fruits, pickles, etc., that have been colored green with copper, and food, especially if acid, that has been cooked or kept in copper vessels, are apt to produce an acute gastro-enteritis. Chronic copper poisoning, so called, is perhaps always due to other substances, as lead or arsenic, and should be treated accordingly.

Antidotes for acute copper poisoning: Encourage vomiting and give albumen (white of egg), which combines with the copper salt to form an insoluble albuminate; or iron filings, which will precipitate the copper in metallic state.

MERCURY is the only metal liquid at ordinary temperatures, and resembles silver in appearance, hence the names hydrargyrum (water silver) and quicksilver (fluid silver). It is so heavy (specific gravity 13.56) that iron and stone float upon it as corks on water. (Fig. 37 represents a marble and a ball of iron floating on mercury.) It does not tarnish in the air unless contaminated with baser metals; dissolves all metals, except iron, to form amalgams.

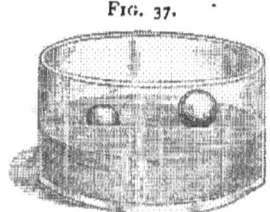

FIG. 37.

Uses.—Metallic mercury is used extensively in the refining of silver and gold, in thermometers and other instruments, with tin in silvering mirrors, and in many other branches of the arts. Metallic mercury, rubbed up with various excipients until globules cease to be visible, forms several officinal preparations. Rubbed with chalk it forms "gray powder," *hydrargyrum cum creta;* with confection of roses and licorice powder it forms "blue pill," *pilula hydrargyri;* and with lard and suet it forms "mercurial ointment," *unguentum hydrargyri*. The therapeutic activity of these preparations is not due to the metallic mercury they contain, but to small quantities of mercurous oxide formed by the oxidation of the finely divided metal. So their strength varies with the thoroughness of the rubbing, the extent of the exposure, and the age of the preparation.

MERCUROUS IODIDE—HgI—*Proto-iodide, Green Iodide, Hydrargyri Iodidum Viride*, U. S. P.—Made by rubbing together chemical equivalents of mercury (200) and iodine (127) until they combine and form a green mass.

MERCURIC IODIDE—HgI$_2$—*Biniodide, Red Iodide, Hydrargyri Iodidum Rubrum.*—Made like the above, except that two equivalents of iodine (twice 127) are employed.

Both the iodides, being insoluble, may be precipitated by adding a solution of KI to a solution of mercurous salt for the one and a mercuric for the other, thus:—

$$HgNO_3 + KI = HgI + KNO_3 \text{ and}$$
$$Hg_2NO_3 + 2KI = HgI_2 + 2KNO_3.$$

The mercuric iodide is dissolved by excess of either the Hg2NO$_3$ or the KI. In precipitating, mercuric iodide is first yellow, but rapidly becomes red. If some of the dry red powder be placed on a sheet of paper and warmed over a lamp, it changes back to yellow, but on shaking or rubbing the red is restored. These changes in color are due to changes in crystalline structure.

MERCUROUS NITRATE—HgNO$_3$—is formed when mercury is treated with cold dilute nitric acid.

MERCURIC NITRATE—Hg2NO$_3$.—*Acid nitrate of mercury* is formed if the mercury be boiled with strong nitric acid. Like all nitrates, both of the above are soluble. It enters into the *liq. hydrargyri nitratis*, U. S. P., and "citrine ointment," *ung. hydrargyri nitratis*, U. S. P.

MERCUROUS SULPHATE—Hg$_2$SO$_4$—is made by digesting sulphuric acid with excess of mercury.

MERCURIC SULPHATE—HgSO$_4$—is made by heating mercury with excess of sulphuric acid. A white, crystalline salt, used in some forms of galvanic batteries. When diluted with water it decomposes into an acid salt, which remains in solution, and a yellow precipitate of oxysulphate, HgSO$_4$.2HgO, called "turpeth mineral," *hydrargyri subsulphas flavus*, U. S. P.

MERCUROUS CHLORIDE—HgCl—*Calomel, mild chloride, Hydrargyri Chloridum Mite*, U. S. P.—is made by heating mercurous sulphate with sodium chloride (Hg$_2$SO$_4$ + 2NaCl = Na$_2$SO$_4$ + 2HgCl), when the mercurous chloride sublimes and is condensed in a cool receiver.

Calomel is a white, insoluble powder. Exposed to light it is slowly decomposed ($2HgCl = Hg + HgCl_2$). With aqua regia, and more slowly with other soluble chlorides, it is converted into mercuric chloride. Calomel probably passes through the stomach unaltered, but is converted into the mercurous oxide by the alkaline fluids in the small intestine.

MERCURIC CHLORIDE—$HgCl_2$—*Bichloride of Mercury, Corrosive Sublimate*—is prepared by sublimation from a mixture of mercuric sulphate and sodium chloride, thus :—

$$HgSO_4 + 2NaCl = Na_2SO_4 + HgCl_2.$$

It is crystalline and soluble, with a disagreeable styptic taste, and is very poisonous; much used in antiseptic surgery.

MERCURIC AMMONIUM CHLORIDE—*Ammoniated Mercury, White Precipitate*, U. S. P.—Formed by adding ammonia to a solution of mercuric chloride; mostly used in ointment. It is a double salt of mercury and NH_2, a derivative of ammonium. Its composition is that of NH_4Cl, in which two atoms of H are displaced by one of Hg, forming NH_2HgCl. The ammonio-sulphate of copper previously described has an analogous composition.

MERCUROUS OXIDE—Hg_2O—*Black Oxide of Mercury*—is made by treating a mercurous salt with a soluble hydrate, as—

$$2HgCl + 2KHO = Hg_2O + 2KCl + H_2O.$$

It is seldom used in medicine.

MERCURIC OXIDE—HgO—*Red or Yellow Oxide.*—When prepared by decomposing mercuric nitrate by heat, it is crystalline and of a red color (*hydrargyri oxidum rubrum*, U. S. P.); but when made by precipitating a mercuric solution with a hydrate,

$$HgCl_2 + 2KHO = HgO + 2KCl + H_2O,$$

it is an amorphous yellow powder (*hydrargyri oxidum flavum*, U. S. P.). The yellow variety, being amorphous and more finely divided, is less gritty and has greater therapeutic activity.

OLEATE OF MERCURY is made by warming the yellow oxide with oleic acid. A liquid or semi-solid. Applied to the skin it is rapidly absorbed.

MERCUROUS SULPHIDE—Hg_2S—is an unstable compound, which

falls as a black precipitate when a mercurous solution is treated with a soluble sulphide.

MERCURIC SULPHIDE—HgS—falls as a black precipitate when a mercuric solution is treated with a soluble sulphide. It is found in nature in crystalline masses called *cinnabar*. By certain processes it may be obtained as a deep-red crystalline powder, called *vermilion*.

Tests.—These consist in adding to the suspected liquid solutions of salts containing radicals capable of uniting with mercury and forming precipitates of the foregoing insoluble compounds. But the *galvanic test* is perhaps the best for clinical purposes. On a gold or copper coin put a drop of the suspected solution acidulated with HCl, and with a piece of baser metal, as a knife blade, touch the coin through the drop of fluid. Mercury, if present, will be deposited on the coin in a silvery film.

Physiological.—*Acute* poisoning occurs from swallowing a single large dose of some of the mercuric compounds, especially corrosive sublimate. The minimum fatal dose of corrosive sublimate is three grains; of white precipitate and turpeth mineral forty grains. Children tolerate mercury much better in proportion to their age than adults. The symptoms are those of severe gastro-enteric irritation. Give albumin, with which it forms an insoluble compound. Iron filings also act as a chemical antidote by decomposing the salt, taking the acidulous radical and depositing the mercury in the metallic state.

Chronic poisoning is often called, from its most prominent symptom, *salivation* or *ptyalism*. It usually occurs from small, but often repeated doses of the mercurous preparations, as blue pill, calomel, etc. One of the first *symptoms* is a delicate red line along the margin of the gums, then comes a metallic taste, abdominal pains, nausea, vomiting, dysenteric diarrhœa, profuse flow of saliva, fetid breath, fever, emaciation, and paralysis. Sphacelation of the mouth and lips sometimes occurs. The *treatment* is to stop the ingestion of poison, and give some astringent, as tannin.

XII. The Silver Group.

SILVER (*Argentum*), ... Ag 108
GOLD (*Aurum*), ... Au 197
PLATINUM, ... Pt 194.4

These are heavy, bright metals, not easily corroded, rare and very valuable. Silver is univalent; gold, trivalent; and platinum, quadrivalent.

SILVER *occurs* free, but often as a sulphide associated with lead in galena. A white, malleable, ductile metal, capable of a high polish; best known conductor of electricity; dissolved readily by nitric, but not by hydrochloric or sulphuric acid, except by the aid of heat; does not tarnish in air unless ozone or H_2S be present.

Used to plate mirrors and articles made of the more corrodible metals; alloyed with copper as coin; for tubes, sutures, etc., in surgery, for it does not corrode and irritate the tissues.

SILVER NITRATE—$AgNO_3$—*Argenti Nitras*, U. S. P., *Lunar Caustic*. *Made* by the action of nitric acid on silver. If coin silver be used, the solution is blue, from the presence of copper. Silver nitrate is a crystalline salt, very soluble. Its taste is acrid, and in large doses it acts as a corrosive poison, destroying the tissues by coagulating their albumin. For use as a cautery it is fused and moulded into sticks.

SILVER OXIDE—Ag_2O—is precipitated as a brown powder on treating a solution of silver nitrate with caustic potash or soda ($2AgNO_3 + 2KHO = 2KNO_3 + Ag_2O + H_2O$). Slightly soluble in water. The other salts of silver are insoluble, and made by precipitating a solution of silver nitrate with a solution containing the appropriate radical.

SILVER CYANIDE—AgCN.

$$AgNO_3 + KCN = AgCN + KNO_3.$$

White precipitate, soluble in ammonium hydrate.

SILVER CHLORIDE—AgCl.*

$$AgNO_3 + NaCl = AgCl + NaNO_3.$$

---

* There are three insoluble chlorides, viz., $PbCl_2$, $HgCl$, and $AgCl$. They may be distinguished by ammonia, which dissolves $AgCl$; blackens $HgCl$, and has no effect on $PbCl_2$.

White precipitate; insoluble in nitric acid, but freely soluble in ammonium hydrate.

SILVER BROMIDE—AgBr.

$$AgNO_3 + KBr = AgBr + KNO_3.$$

Yellowish-white precipitate; slightly soluble in ammonium hydrate.

SILVER IODIDE—AgI.

$$AgNO_3 + KI = AgI + KNO_3.$$

Yellow precipitate; insoluble in ammonium hydrate.

Effects of Light.—Light decomposes salts of silver, especially if organic matter be present, depositing metallic silver in a fine, black powder, hence their uses in photography, and in making indelible inks, hair dyes, etc. The black stain of silver on the hands or clothes may be removed by potassium cyanide or by applying tincture of iodine and washing in ammonia-water. When persons have taken silver salts for a long time, it sometimes occurs that the tissues, especially the skin, are permanently darkened. This is due to the decomposition of the silver salt under the influence of organic matter and light.

Poisoning occurs mostly from swallowing the nitrate, which is the only soluble silver salt. It is a severe corrosive poison, destroying the tissues by coagulating their albumin. Its best antidote is a soluble chloride, as common salt, which forms the insoluble silver chloride. Albumin is also a good antidote.

GOLD *occurs* widely, but sparingly distributed; always free, mixed with sand and quartz, from which it is separated by agitation with water or by dissolving it out with mercury. It is a soft, bright, yellow metal; so malleable that it may be beaten into sheets (gold-leaf) less than one two-hundred-thousandth of an inch in thickness. These transmit green light. For coinage and general use gold is usually hardened by the addition of copper or silver, the amount of which is indicated by the term *carat fine*. Thus, pure gold is twenty-four carat, and eighteen, sixteen, and twelve carat signify so many twenty-fourths of pure gold.

Gold does not tarnish in the air; is unaffected by any single acid, but nitro-muriatic acid (aqua regia) easily dissolves it, forming *auric chloride*, AuCl₃, a caustic salt, which is sometimes given as a nerve tonic and aphrodisiac. Dose, one-twentieth to one-tenth of a grain.

PLATINUM, *occurs* free, associated with the allied metals, palladium, rhodium, ruthinium and iridium. Owing to its scarcity it is almost as costly as gold. Resembles silver in appearance; can be melted only with very great difficulty, and very few substances corrode it; hence it is used to make vessels that are to be exposed to very high heat or to contain corrosive chemicals. Platinum wire is also used in flame testing.

Platinum readily dissolves in nitro-muriatic acid, forming *platinic chloride*, PtCl₄, a valuable reagent for potassium, ammonium and alkaloids.

In the table of the elements are given the names, symbols and atomic weights of many substances that are as yet of little or no medical interest, and have therefore not received special description. They are rare elements, widely distributed but in minute quantities. Some of them are of considerable scientific interest. Molybdenum, as ammonium molybdate, forms a valuable test-reagent for phosphoric acid. Osmium, as osmic acid, OsO₄, is used in microscopy.

TABLE.—TO DETERMINE THE METALLIC RADICAL OF A SALT IN AQUEOUS OR SLIGHTLY ACID SOLUTION BY SYSTEMATIC ANALYSIS.

Add hydrochloric acid.

Precipitate
Hg (ous) Pb Ag.
Collect, wash, and add NH_4HO.
Hg ppt., blackened.
Pb ppt., still white.
Ag ppt., dissolved.
Sb and Bi may also be precipitated by HCl, but are dissolved on adding more HCl.

If HCl gave no precipitate the metal is still in the liquid; pass H_2S through the solution.

Precipitate
Cd Cu Hg(ic) Pb Bi As Sb Sn
Au Pt.
Collect, wash, add NH_4HS.
Insoluble. Soluble.
Cd, yellow
Cu   } black.
Hg(ic)
Pb
Bi

As (ous) & ic } yellow.
Sn (ic)

Sb, orange.

Sn (ous)
Au   } black.
Pt

Apply special tests for each to the original solution. For these, see the previous pages.

If H_2S gave no precipitate add NH_4Cl, NH_3HO and NH_4HS.

Precipitate
Zn Mn CO Ni Al
Fe Cr
Zn } white.
Al
Cr, green.
Mn, skin-tint.
Ni } black.
Co
Fe

Test specially for each in original solution.
See previous pages.

If NH_4HS gave no precipitate add $(NH_4)_2CO_3$.

Precipitate
Ba Sr Ca
Collect, wash, dissolve in $HC_2H_3O_2$, add K_2CrO_4.

Sol. Sr Ca.
Add dil. H_2SO_4.

Ppt. Ba.

Ppt. Sr.—Ca.

If $(NH_4)_2CO_3$ gave no precipitate add $(NH_4)_2HAsO_4$.

Ppt. Mg.

If no precipitate, test original solution in flame on loop of Pt wire.
Li, crimson.
Na, yellow.
K, violet.
If neither, test orig. sol. for NH_4.

PART I.—INORGANIC CHEMISTRY.

TABLE.—TO DETERMINE THE ACIDULOUS (NEGATIVE) RADICAL OF AN ORDINARY SALT IN AQUEOUS SOLUTION, POUR SMALL PORTIONS INTO FIVE TEST-TUBES, THE SOLUTION RENDERED NEUTRAL, IF NECESSARY, BY AMMONIA. THEN ADD TO EACH RESPECTIVELY A FEW DROPS OF SULPHURIC ACID, BARIUM CHLORIDE, CALCIUM CHLORIDE, SILVER NITRATE, AND FERRIC CHLORIDE. INTERPRET THEIR EFFECTS ACCORDING TO THE FOLLOWING TABLE:

H_2SO_4 decomposes	$BaCl_2$ precipitates	$CaCl_2$ precipitates	$AgNO_3$ precipitates	Fe_2Cl_6 precipitates	Not precipitated.
Sulphides Sulphites Carbonates { With effervescence of H_2S and SO_2 known by smell, and CO_2 having no noticeable odor.	(All white.) Sulphates, insol. in HCl. Sulphites } Effervesce with acids. Carbonates Citrates } Char when heated on platinum oil. Tartrates Borates, Oxalates, Phosphates.	(All white.) Sulphates, sol. in much water. Borates } soluble in NH_4Cl. Carbonates Citrates Phosphates. Oxalates. Sulphites. Tartrates.	Borates Carbonates Chlorates Citrates Cyanides Oxalates Sulphates Tartrates } white. Bromides } yellowish-white. Iodides } yellow. Phosphates Sulphides, black.	Phosphates } yellowish-white. Borates, yellowish. Oxalates, yellow. Carbonates, reddish. Acetates, red if neutral. Sulphides, black.	Nitrates. Chlorates. Apply special tests. (see previous pages.)
Cyanides with odor of HCN.		All sol. in acetic acid, except oxalate and some sulphate and tartrate. All sol. in HCl, except much sulphate. Citrate and tartrate char when heated on platinum foil. Carbonate and sulphite effervesce with acids, evolving H_2S and SO_2.	All soluble in dilute nitric acid, except chloride, bromide, iodide, cyanide, and sulphide.		
Acetates with odor of acetic acid, especially if warmed.					

TABLE.—THE SOLUBILITY OR INSOLUBILITY OF SALTS IN WATER.

Much time may be saved by not applying special tests to an aqueous solution for salts known to be insoluble in water.

S, soluble; Ss, slightly soluble; I, insoluble; ?, unknown or does not exist.

PART II.—ORGANIC CHEMISTRY.

Formerly organic chemistry was defined as the chemistry of the compounds produced only by organized life. Gradually this definition has been abandoned, for with the increase of chemical knowledge many substances identical with the animal and vegetable products have of late years been made in the laboratory without the aid of the vital force, and probably, if their chemical constitution were fully understood, all animal and vegetable products could be duplicated artificially. However, chemistry has not, and probably never will, produce an *organized* body, *i. e.*, one having an anatomical, cellular structure.

It is a noticeable fact that every organic compound contains carbon. Hence, *organic chemistry* is now defined to be "the chemistry of the carbon compounds," and the following pages may be considered a resumption of the study of that element.

Though carbon forms compounds of infinite number and extreme complexity, it is with the aid of a very few other elements, viz.: hydrogen, oxygen, nitrogen, and occasionally sulphur, phosphorus and iron—sometimes others; but the larger number of even the artificial compounds contain only the above-named elements. This is due to the fact that the carbon atoms possess, in the highest degree, the power of *combining with each other and interchanging valences,* forming groups or chains around which the other elements are arranged. But for this power carbon could form only one saturated compound with hydrogen, CH_4. Carbon being quadrivalent, the compounds C_2H_6 and C_3H_8 would be unsaturated. Experiment, however, proves that they are saturated compounds. The explanation is that the carbon atoms combine with each other, mutually neutralizing one or more valences, thus:—

$$H-\overset{\overset{H}{|}}{\underset{\underset{H}{|}}{C}}-H; \quad H-\overset{\overset{H}{|}}{\underset{\underset{H}{|}}{C}}-\overset{\overset{H}{|}}{\underset{\underset{H}{|}}{C}}-H; \quad H-\overset{\overset{H}{|}}{\underset{\underset{H}{|}}{C}}-\overset{\overset{H}{|}}{\underset{\underset{H}{|}}{C}}-\overset{\overset{H}{|}}{\underset{\underset{H}{|}}{C}}-H.$$

It will be observed that these formulæ have a common difference of CH_2. They are said to form a *homologous series*. When the carbon remains the same but the hydrogen differs by H_2, the series is said to be *isologous*.

In the following examples each vertical column represents a homologous, each horizontal line an isologous series:—

CH_4	CH_2	C
C_2H_6	C_2H_4	C_2H_2
C_3H_8	C_3H_6	C_3H_4
C_4H_{10}	C_4H_8	C_4H_6
C_5H_{12}	C_5H_{10}	C_5H_8
etc.	etc.	etc.

Without this arrangement in series, it would be impossible to remember the composition of organic substances.

In systematic works on organic chemistry, these series form the basis of classification; but as this necessitates mentioning thousands of bodies of no medical interest, it would be impracticable in a work like this. We shall therefore adopt the following :—

Hydrocarbons and their derivatives.
Alcohols.
Ethers (including oils and fats).
Aldehydes.
Organic acids.
Carbohydrates (sugars and starches).
Glucosides.
Ammonium substitutions.
Natural alkaloids.

Hydrocarbons are compounds of carbon with hydrogen. Of these CH_4* is the type from which all the other members of this class may be regarded as derived in isologous or homologous series. *Petroleum* is a mixture of the homologous derivatives from the first (CH_4) to about the sixteenth ($C_{16}H_{34}$). These are separated by distilling the crude oil. Those having the smallest molecules, being

---

* CH_4, *methane, marsh gas* or *light carburetted hydrogen*, is a constituent of coal (illuminating) gas, and is also formed by the decomposition of vegetable matter under water, as in marshes. It occurs sometimes in coal mines (fire damp) where, mixed with air, it causes fearful explosions. Made in laboratory by heating a mixture of four parts each of sodium acetate and sodium hydrate with six parts of lime in powder. It is colorless, almost odorless, and not poisonous.

PART II.—ORGANIC CHEMISTRY. 99

lightest, pass over first, forming *naphtha, benzine*, etc.* As the heat is increased the medium-weight compounds come over next, forming *kerosene*. The residuum consists of the heaviest carbohydrides, which can be distilled only by high heat, forming *lubricating oil, vaseline, paraffine*, etc. All the lighter products are liable to give off vapors which, mixing with air, are explosive. In most States it is illegal to sell kerosene which gives off an inflammable vapor ("flashes") below 100° F.

The TURPENE series begins with tritone, C_3H_2, but it is the eighth member, $C_{10}H_{16}$, that is of medical interest, for this represents the composition of most of the *volatile* or *essential oils*. These various oils (of lemon, orange, cloves, pepper, lavender, bergamot, etc.), though having differences in chemical and physical properties, all have the same composition, $C_{10}H_{16}$.

Such bodies are said to be *isomeric* (ἴσος, equal, μέρος, part).

Volatile oils are found in plants, especially the flowers, of which they are usually the odorous essences (hence called also *essential oils*). Obtained by distillation from flowers, etc. Very slightly soluble in water (*aquæ*), but quite soluble in alcohol (*spiritus*). A cologne is an alcoholic solution of an assortment of volatile oils.

Turpentine (*oleum terebinthinæ*, U. S. P.) is the most important of the volatile oils, and may be taken as a type of the class. It is a thin, colorless liquid, a valuable solvent of oils and resins; absorbs oxygen and stores it up as ozone, gaining thereby oxidizing, antiseptic, and disinfectant properties. By the action of concentrated sulphuric acid, turpentine is changed into *terebene* ($C_{10}H_{16}$), a valuable remedy for bronchitis and flatulence.

On exposure to air the turpenes oxidize with the production of resins and camphors.

RESINS are a numerous class, many of which are true acids. Soluble

* Rhigoline	boils at	32° F.,	used as spray for anæsthesia.
Gasoline	"	119° F.,	" for making "air gas."
Naphtha	"	220° F.,	" " dissolving fats and rubber.
Benzene	"	300° F.,	" " varnishes and paints.
Kerosene	"	350° F.,	" " ordinary lamps.
Mineral sperm oil	"	425° F.,	" " lubricating machinery.
Lubricating oil	"	575° F.,	" " " "
Petrolatum, U. S. P.,	semi-solid,	" " ointments.
Paraffine,	solid,	" " candles, etc.

in alcohol but insoluble in water, except by the intervention of an alkali, with which they will unite to form soluble soaps.

The officinal resin (*resína*, U. S. P.) is formed by the oxidation of turpentine as it exudes from the pine tree.

Solutions of shellac, mastic, copal and others are used as varnishes. In the natural state resins are usually mixed with other substances.* Mixed with volatile oils they form *oleo-resins* and *balsams, e.g.*, benzoin, tolu, and balsam of Peru, and with gums, *gum-resins, e.g.*, ammoniac, myrrh and asafœtida.

CAMPHORS.—*Common camphor*—$C_{10}H_{16}O$—obtained from the camphor laurel, is a white, crystalline, volatile solid of a peculiar pungent order; slightly soluble in water (*aqua camphoræ*, U. S. P.), and freely soluble in alcohol (*tinct. camphoræ*) and ether.

Monobromated camphor—$C_{10}H_{15}BrO$—used in medicine as a sedative, is formed by substituting one atom of bromine for one of hydrogen in ordinary camphor.

Menthol is a camphor-like body found in oil of peppermint, and possesses the odor of that plant.

Caoutchouc, or *India-rubber*, and *gutta-percha* are inspissated juices of certain tropical trees. Caoutchouc is elastic; gutta-percha is not.

---

* PROXIMATE AND ULTIMATE PRINCIPLES.—Most organic bodies in their natural state are mixtures of several different substances. These substances that naturally exist, mixed together to form a body, are called its *proximate principles*. The separation of these unaltered is called *proximate analysis*. Different methods must be devised for different substances. For example: Take a piece of vegetable tissue containing woody fibre, starch, sugar, resin, and volatile oil. The oil is removed by a gentle heat; the resin is dissolved out by alcohol; the sugar by cold water, and the starch by boiling in water, leaving the woody fibre.

The *ultimate principles* of a body are the elements (carbon, hydrogen, etc.) of which it is composed, and the recognition and measuring of these is *ultimate analysis*. This, while requiring careful manipulation, is simple in principle. The body is burned with a full supply of oxygen, converting the carbon into CO_2 and the hydrogen into H_2O. These are collected and weighed, and the quantities of carbon and hydrogen in them are calculated. The amount of oxygen, if any, is determined by subtracting the sum of the carbon and hydrogen from the weight of the original body. For example: 46 grains of alcohol (C, H and O) burned completely makes:—

    88 grains of CO_2 equivalent to 24 grains of C.
    54 grains of H_2O equivalent to 6 grains of H.
    46 grains alcohol, minus 30 grains (24 + 6), = 16 grains of O.

The less common elements, chlorine, nitrogen, sulphur, phosphorus, etc., are determined by special methods.

Both are hardened (vulcanized) by combining with sulphur. They are unaffected by most chemicals and solvents. Chloroform is their best solvent.

Alcohols.—*The Alcohol Radicals* are a homologous series of univalent basylous radicals, so called because they are the bases of the most important alcohols. Their compounds are numerous, and enter largely into the *materia medica*. In the following table a few of these compounds are given :—

Radicals.	Alcohols (Hydrates).	Oxides, Ethers.	Examples of Compound Ethers.		Aldehydes.	Acids.
			Nitrates.	Sulphates.		
Methyl, CH_3	CH_3HO	$(CH_3)_2O$	CH_3NO_3	$(CH_3)_2SO_4$	CH_2O	CH_2O_2
Ethyl, C_2H_5	C_2H_5HO	$(C_2H_5)_2O$	$C_2H_5NO_3$	$(C_2H_5)_2SO_4$	C_2H_4O	$C_2H_4O_2$
Propyl, C_3H_7	C_3H_7HO	$(C_3H_7)_2O$	$C_3H_7NO_3$	$(C_3H_7)_2SO_4$	C_3H_6O	$C_3H_6O_2$
Butyl, C_4H_9	C_4H_9HO	$(C_4H_9)_2O$	$C_4H_9NO_3$	$(C_4H_9)_2SO_4$	C_4H_8O	$C_4H_8O_2$
Amyl, C_5H_{11}	$C_5H_{11}HO$	$(C_5H_{11})_2O$	$C_5H_{11}NO_3$	$(C_5H_{11})_2SO_4$	$C_5H_{10}O$	$C_5H_{10}O_2$
Hexyl, C_6H_{13}	$C_6H_{13}HO$	$(C_6H_{13})_2O$	$C_6H_{13}NO_3$	$(C_6H_{13})_2SO_4$	$C_6H_{12}O$	$C_6H_{12}O_2$
etc.	etc.	etc.	etc.	etc.	etc.	etc.

In the formation of these compounds the starting-point is not the radicals, but their hydrates, the alcohols. When an alcohol is oxidized with a limited supply of oxygen, two atoms of hydrogen are removed and no oxygen is added. This forms the *aldehyde*, thus :—

Methyl   Methyl
Alcohol.   Aldehyde.
$$CH_3HO + O = CH_2O + H_2O.$$

If there is a full oxidation, an atom of oxygen takes the place of the two atoms of hydrogen removed, and forms the corresponding acid, as—

Methyl   Formic
Alcohol.   Acid.
$$CH_3HO + O_2 = CH_2O_2 + H_2O.$$

In the formation of aldehydes and acids the radical supplies part of the hydrogen removed and loses its identity. As part of the hydrogen in an acid forms the positive radical, it is written first ; *e. g.*, formic acid is written $HCHO_2$, instead of CH_2O_2. The various other compounds of these radicals are called *ethers ;* the oxides being called *simple ethers*, the others *compound ethers*. They are generally formed by treating the appropriate alcohol with the appropriate acid.

METHYLIC ALCOHOL—CH_3HO—*Wood Naphtha, Wood Spirit,*

Wood Alcohol, Pyroligneous Spirit, Methyl Hydrate—does not exist in nature. Made by the destructive distillation of wood. The commercial article has a very disagreeable odor and taste from the presence of tarry matters, etc.; but when pure, methylic alcohol resembles ordinary alcohol in its properties and physiological action. It is not used in medicine, but is extensively employed in the arts as a solvent, as in the preparation of varnishes, etc.

Methylated spirit is ordinary alcohol to which has been added one-tenth part of commercial methylic alcohol to render it unfit for drinking, and thus relieve it of the heavy tax imposed upon alcoholic beverages.

ETHYLIC ALCOHOL—C_2H_5HO—*Ethyl Hydrate, Spirits of Wine, Vinic Alcohol, Alcohol.*—Alcohol does not exist in nature, but is produced in a number of reactions. Liquids containing it (wines, etc.) have been known from the remotest antiquity, and are obtained by allowing liquids containing glucose (grape sugar) to ferment.

$$\underset{\text{Glucose.}}{C_6H_{12}O_6} = \underset{\text{Alcohol.}}{2C_2H_5HO} + \underset{\text{Carbon Dioxide.}}{2CO_2}.$$

The alcohol is then separated by distillation, for, being more volatile than the water, it passes over first.

Commercial alcohol always contains water, and when pure or *absolute* alcohol is required, the commercial article is mixed with some substance which is very avid of water, as quicklime, and then again distilled.

Alcohol is a light, colorless liquid, of a pleasant, pungent odor and burning taste. Has a great affinity for water, which probably accounts for its preserving animal tissues and coagulating albumin.

It is largely used in the arts and in pharmacy, principally as a solvent, but also in the manufacture of various substances, as vinegar, chloral, chloroform, iodoform,* ether, etc.; and as a fuel when a hot and smokeless flame is needed; and as a menstruum in the preparation of tinctures and spirits.

Alcoholic solutions of fixed medicinal substances are called *tinctures;* those of volatile principles, *spirits.*

Alcohol is employed in various forms and degrees of concentration.

---

* **Experiment.**—To test for alcohol in a solution: Warm; add a few scales of iodine, and then caustic potash until the color is discharged. On cooling, yellow scales of iodoform are deposited.

Absolute alcohol is rarely employed. *Alcohol fortius*, U.S.P., stronger alcohol, contains 92 per cent. of alcohol. *Alcohol*, U. S. P., is the ordinary rectified spirit, and contains 85 per cent. of alcohol. *Alcohol dilutum*, U. S. P., diluted alcohol, is made by mixing water and alcohol, equal parts.

Spiritus frumenti, U. S. P., whisky, and *spiritus vini gallici*, U. S. P., brandy, are obtained by distillation; the former from fermented grain, and the latter from fermented grape juice. They contain about 50 per cent. of alcohol. They are colored by the addition of caramel (burnt sugar). Their flavor is due to small quantities of other alcohols produced in the fermentation, and to certain ethers formed from these alcohols, especially as the liquor "*ages*."

A large class of alcoholic beverages are made by fermenting various liquids containing sugar or some substance capable of conversion into sugar.

Beer, ale and *porter* are infusions of malted grain, fermented and flavored with hops. They therefore contain the soluble constituents of the grain. Their alcoholic strength is about 5 per cent. *Wines* are prepared by allowing grape juice to ferment. The alcoholic strength of the different varieties varies from 10 to 25 per cent. Sherry (*vinum Xericum*) and port (*vinum rubrum*) are the only ones officinal. *Cider* is the fermented juice of the apple, prepared very much in the same way as wine is from grape juice, and contains about 5 per cent. of alcohol. It is very prone to acetous fermentation and liable to produce colic and diarrhœa.

Alcohol, when concentrated, abstracts water from the tissues and coagulates their albuminoid constituents, and is a poison. In full doses (*always best with food*) it produces a sense of warmth in the stomach, general comfort and exhilaration, followed by incoherence of ideas and impairment of muscular coördination. Taken habitually, in any of its forms, it impairs the mental and moral force of its victim and produces in the various organs, especially the liver and kidneys, the degenerative changes characteristic of chronic alcoholism. It should never be taken in health, but as a medicine it is the most valuable of stimulants. In cases of acute poisoning by alcohol, the stomach and bladder should be evacuated, and the depression (coma) counteracted by strong coffee, the cold douche, and other stimulants.

AMYLIC ALCOHOL—$C_5H_{11}HO$—*Amyl Hydrate, Fusel Oil.*—This is a heavy liquid, soluble in alcohol but not in water, hence incorrectly called an oil. It is produced in the fermentation of grain and potatoes, and is the most deleterious impurity in common whisky before it has undergone the refining process.

It has a penetrating, disagreeable odor, resembling that of mean whisky. Although not fragrant itself, its ethers, when dissolved in ethylic alcohol, have the taste and odor of various fruits, and are used in the preparations of artificial fruit essences.*

The other alcohols of this series are of no medical interest.

GLYCERYLIC ALCOHOL—C_3H_53HO—*Glycerine*.—Being made from fats in the manufacture of soaps and candles, it has been called (Scheele, 1779) the "sweet principle of fats"; but it has no chemical analogy to them, being the hydrate of the trivalent radical glyceryl, C_3H_5, and therefore an alcohol. It is a colorless, odorless, sweet, viscid liquid, avid of water, neutral in reaction; a solvent of a great many mineral and organic substances (*glycerites*), ranking in this respect next to alcohol and water. Glycerine is used in medicine mainly as a solvent and as a local application.

Nitroglycerine—$C_3H_5(NO_3)_3$—is formed by treating glycerine with nitric acid. It is an oily liquid and one of the most dangerous of explosives. Mixed with fine silica (sand) it is dynamite.

In medicine nitroglycerine is used as a heart stimulant.

PHENYL ALCOHOL—C_6H_5HO—*Phenol—Carbolic Acid*.—This is an alcohol, the hydrate of phenyl, C_6H_5, a radical of the aromatic series, but is called an acid because it combines with bases and forms bodies resembling salts (carbolates or phenates).

Carbolic acid is formed in a number of reactions, but the commercial article is obtained exclusively from coal tar. It has a strong, disagreeable odor; occurs as white crystals, which melt on the addition of a small quantity of water; reddens by age; slightly soluble in water, but very soluble in glycerine, the solution being soluble in water; stains skin and mucous membranes white by coagulating their albumin; and is a corrosive poison. Albumin is its best antidote.

Carbolic acid is a powerful antiseptic and disinfectant. Applied locally it is astringent, sedative, and even anæsthetic.

---

* **Experiment.**—To a half drachm of fusel oil in a test-tube add some sodium or potassium acetate and a few drops of sulphuric acid. Warm the mixture, and the acetate of amyl (essence of pear) may be recognized by its odor.

PART II.—ORGANIC CHEMISTRY. 105

Carbolic acid and sulphuric acid will combine to form sulphocarbolic acid (phenyl bisulphate, $C_6H_5HSO_4$). Sodium sulphocarbolate, U. S. P., is a soluble salt sometimes used in medicine.

Resorcin—($C_6H_4$2HO).—Closely related to phenol, but a stronger antiseptic and much less poisonous. It occurs in soluble, colorless, odorless crystals of a sweetish taste. It is given as an antizymotic in diseases attended with fermentative changes and in the specific fevers.

Creasote is a complex mixture obtained from wood tar; closely allied to carbolic acid in its properties and uses, but may be readily distinguished from it by being insoluble in glycerine.

One of the constituents of creasote is *guiacol*, of late used as an inhalation in phthisis.

MANNITYL ALCOHOL—$C_6H_6$6HO—*Mannite*.—This is the principal ingredient in manna, a white, gummy substance exuding from certain trees. Mannite is a crystalline substance closely resembling glucose, except that it does not undergo the vinous fermentation, and does not respond to Trommer's or Fehling's tests.

Ethers.—The *simple* ethers (oxides) are the results of dehydrating two molecules of alcohol by means of sulphuric acid; the *compound* ethers are made by treating the appropriate alcohol with the appropriate acid.

ETHYL OXIDE—$(C_2H_5)_2O$—*Sulphuric Ether, Ether.*—Ether is made by distilling a mixture of alcohol and sulphuric acid; * hence, the misnomer, *sulphuric ether.*

A small quantity of sulphuric acid is capable of converting a large amount of alcohol into ether, for it is unaltered in the reaction; in fact, the process might go on indefinitely but for the acid being so diluted with the water derived from the alcohol, as to finally stop the reaction. The sulphuric acid is said to act by its mere presence, by *catalysis;* or, in other words, it acts because it acts, a ready but feminine way of explaining many otherwise inexplicable chemical and physiological phenomena.

---

* **Experiment.**—Into a large test-tube pour alcohol and half as much sulphuric acid; warm and note the odor of the ether evolved. Next adapt a cork with delivery tube, and slowly distill the ether into a cool test-tube. By adding more alcohol the operation may be repeated again and again.

8

The true rationale is as follows:—

And then
$$C_2H_5HO + H_2SO_4 = C_2H_5HSO_4 + H_2O.$$
$$C_2H_5HSO_4 + C_2H_5HO = (C_2H_5)_2O + H_2SO_4.$$

Ether is a colorless, very volatile liquid, of a peculiar odor, called *ethereal*. It burns easily, and its vapor, mixed with air or oxygen, explodes when ignited; * so ether should never be used near, especially above, a flame. Ether is a valuable solvent, and, as it evaporates very rapidly, it is used to produce cold.† But its chief use in medicine is as an anæsthetic. Being less liable to paralyze the nerve centres, it is safer than chloroform.

ETHYL CHLORIDE—C_2H_5Cl.—*Hydrochloric ether* must not be confounded with the so-called *chloric ether*, which is an alcoholic solution of chloroform.

ETHYL BROMIDE—C_2H_5Br—*Hydrobromic Ether.*—A valuable anæsthetic, but not much used.

ETHYL NITRITE—$C_2H_5NO_2$—*Nitrous Ether.*—If nitric acid be treated with copper or starch it loses part of its oxygen, being converted into nitrous acid (HNO_2), which will unite with alcohol, forming nitrous ether and water, thus:—

$$C_2H_5HO + HNO_2 = C_2H_5NO_2 + H_2O.$$

Nitrous ether is a yellowish liquid, of an apple-like odor and sweetish taste. It is used only diluted with alcohol, forming the *spiritus ætheris nitrosi*, U. S. P., commonly called *sweet spirits of nitre*.

AMYL NITRITE—$C_5H_{11}NO_2$.—Made like ethyl nitrite, except that amylic alcohol is used. Nitrite of amyl is a volatile, oily liquid, of a peculiar odor, resembling that of bananas. It is given by inhalation, especially in epilepsy, for which purpose it is put up in glass bulbs holding about two drops. These are crushed and inhaled during the *aura*.

CHLOROFORM—*Trichlormethane.*—Methyl, having only one free

---

* **Experiment.**—Put a drachm of ether in a dish and apply a flame. The vapor, mixed with air, explodes; the rest burns rapidly.

† **Experiment.**—Set a test-tube of water in a beaker of ether. Blow air briskly through the ether; the water will freeze.

valence, must give up two atoms of its hydrogen in order to combine with three atoms of chlorine, making the formula of chloroform $CHCl_3$. This is the most used of all the ethers. Chloroform is made by distilling a mixture of chlorinated lime, water, and ordinary alcohol, but of late is being made by a patented process from acetone, which, being a by-product in certain technical operations, is very cheap. It is a colorless, volatile liquid, of a pleasant ethereal odor and sweet taste. It is heavier than water, and does not dissolve in it, but is soluble in alcohol and ether; not easily ignited; a good solvent for phosphorus, iodine, India-rubber, and the alkaloids. Chloroform is sometimes given by the stomach as a sedative, but most frequently administered by inhalation as an anæsthetic, for which purpose it should be of undoubted purity. Pure chloroform is not colored by an equal volume of pure sulphuric acid, nor should its specific gravity be below 1.480.

If chloroform be taken by the stomach, it being insoluble, is absorbed very slowly; and its principal action is the local irritation of the mucous surfaces. Recovery has followed a dose of four ounces, and death has been caused by one drachm taken into the stomach. The vapor acts more energetically, and seems to owe its potency for evil to its paralyzing influence on the nerve centres, especially those of the heart. So chloroform vapor should never be administered except by a capable physician, and well diluted with atmosphere. However, death has occurred from the inhalation of moderate quantities of chloroform properly diluted, and at the hands of careful physicians, and the autopsy revealed no heart lesion.

There is no chemical antidote for chloroform. When it has been swallowed, evacuate the stomach; when inhaled, lower the head, give fresh air, employ artificial respiration, and apply the induced current.

The poison is usually recognized by its odor.

IODOFORM—CHI_3.—Made by the action of iodine and potash on alcohol; yellow scales; insoluble in water, and of a saffron-like odor, which is the chief objection to its use. Light decomposes it, giving it a violet color. Iodoform is used on ulcers, etc., as an anæsthetic, alterative and antiseptic.

FIXED OILS AND FATS.—These are ethers—combinations of glyceryl (C_3H_6) with oleic, stearic, butyric, palmitic, and other fat acids. The natural fats are mixtures of these.* Those containing mostly oleate of glyceryl (olein) are liquid. Warm-blooded animals yield mostly solid; cold-blooded, liquid fats. Drying oils are such as absorb oxygen from the air and become resinous, *e. g.*, linseed. Many fats partially decompose on exposure, producing free acid, and become *rancid*. The fixed oils are insoluble in water, soluble in alcohol, ether and chloroform.

The compounds of the fatty acids with the metals of the alkalies (K, Na, NH_4, etc.), are soluble and are called *soaps*. The soaps formed with the other metallic radicals are insoluble and usually called *plasters*. Lead plaster is officinal. Soaps are made by the *saponification* of a fat with a caustic alkali. For example :—

Stearine. Sodium Stearate. Glycerine.
$$(C_3H_5)(C_{18}H_{32}O_2)_3 + 3NaHO = 3NaC_{18}H_{35}O_2 + C_3H_5(HO)_3.$$

When soap dissolves in cold water, it decomposes into an acid salt which makes the soapsuds and a small quantity of free alkali which does the cleaning.

Aldehydes.—An unimportant class. They constitute the first step in the oxidation of alcohols into acids, viz., the removal of hydrogen (hence the name). Since nothing has taken the place of the hydrogen removed, they are unsaturated and very prone to change, especially to take on oxygen and form the acids.

ETHYL ALDEHYDE, *acetic aldehyde*, or simply *aldehyde*† (C_2H_4O), is a colorless, volatile, acid liquid of a pungent odor. One of its modifications, called *paraldehyde*, is used as a hypnotic, which unlike morphine is followed by no unpleasant effects, except a pungent odor to the breath, and, unlike chloral, does not affect the heart. Dose, ʒss–ʒj.

CHLORAL.—If chlorine displace three atoms of hydrogen in ethyl aldehyde, it forms *tri-chlor-aldehyde*, or chloral (C_2HCl_3O), a colorless,

---

* In "lanolin," the fat obtained from sheeps' wool, the fat acids are combined not with glycerine, but with *cholesterine*, $C_{26}H_{43}HO$, an excrementitious principle of animal bodies. It is a very absorbable base for ointments.

† Experiment.—To a little bichromate and sulphuric acid mixture in a test-tube add a little alcohol; or hold a hot glass rod in a beaker containing a little ether. The peculiar pungent odor is that of aldehyde.

heavy liquid. With a molecule of water this forms a white crystalline solid, called *chloral hydrate*, having a pungent but agreeable odor and taste. Warmed with an alkali it decomposes, thus :—

Chloral. Sod. Formate. Chloroform.
$$C_2HCl_3O + NaHO = NaCHO_2 + CHCl_3.$$

Liebreich thought this reaction would occur in the warm alkaline blood and the sedative action of chloroform be obtained. Though mistaken in this, he found chloral hydrate a valuable hypnotic. The chloral habit is difficult to cure. In overdoses chloral is a poison, and cases are multiplying as its powers become better known. No chemical antidote. Evacuate the stomach, give stimulants, and maintain the respiration and bodily warmth.

Organic Acids.—These are regarded by chemists as the natural results of the oxidation of alcohols. But as most of them were discovered before their relation to the alcohols was known, their names often have no connection with those of the alcohols. We take up only the most important.

ACETIC ACID.—$HC_2H_3O_2$.—This is the acid of vinegar. Formed in a great many reactions, but made mainly by the destructive distillation of wood, or by the oxidation of ordinary alcohol. If wine, cider, or other alcoholic liquors be exposed to the air, a fungus (*mycoderma aceti*) forms on the surface and acts as an oxygen carrier, and the alcohol is converted into acetic acid, thus :—

$$C_2H_5HO + O_2 = HC_2H_3O_2 + H_2O.$$

A more rapid process is to pass the alcohol through barrels filled with beech shavings.

Acetic acid is a colorless liquid, of a pungent, sour taste and smell. When free from water (glacial) it crystallizes at temperatures below 60° F. Acetic acid in dilute solution (vinegar) is much used for domestic purposes. For medicinal use the crude vinegar is purified by distillation, forming *acidum aceticum dilutum*, U. S. P.

As all the acetates are soluble, their best test is to add a strong acid and recognize the acetic acid set free, by its odor.

BENZOIC ACID exists in many balsams and gum-resins. When benzoin is heated benzoic acid sublimes in silky needles of a pleasant balsamic odor. Or, if the urine of herbivorous animals be boiled with hydrochloric acid, the hippuric acid is converted into benzoic acid. But the acid obtained from this source may be known by its urinous odor. It is now made by the oxidation of benzene, the principal constituent of coal-tar.

CARBAZOTIC or PICRIC ACID is a yellow substance, of a bitter taste, made by the action of nitric acid on carbolic acid. Used in the arts as a yellow dye.

CARBOLIC ACID.—Already described among alcohols.

CITRIC ACID exists in the juices of many fruits, especially the lemon. Forms colorless crystals which are very soluble, and possess a sour taste. Many of its salts are used in medicine.

FORMIC ACID—$HCHO_2$—is the oxidation product of methylic alcohol. It was formerly obtained from the red ant (*formica rufa*), but now made artificially. It exists in stinging nettle, pine needles, etc., and also in the stings of most insects.

GALLIC ACID.—When galls are moistened and exposed to the action of the atmosphere, the tannic acid they contain is converted into gallic acid. It resembles tannic acid, but may be distinguished by its not precipitating a solution of gelatin.

LACTIC ACID (*lactis*, of milk).—This is the acid of sour milk, where it is formed by the fermentation of the sugar of milk through the agency of the casein. It is also formed in the body by the decomposition of glucose, thus:—

$$C_6H_{12}O_6 = 2H_2C_3H_4O_3.$$

It is a syrupy liquid, of a very sour taste.

MALIC ACID (*malum*, an apple) exists in many fruits, as apples, cherries, etc., and very abundantly in garden rhubarb.

OXALIC ACID—$H_2C_2O_4$.—The acid and its salts are found in many plants, especially the sorrel (oxalis) grasses. In certain pathological conditions it is formed in the body and eliminated in the urine as calcium oxalate. It is made in large quantities by the action of nitric acid on sugar, or of alkalies on sawdust. Oxalic acid closely resembles Epsom salts, for which it is sometimes taken by mistake. It is a powerful irritant poison. Being cheap and largely used for removing ink stains, cleaning copper, etc., poisoning by oxalic acid is by no means rare. Its best antidote is chalk, or some other compound of calcium, with which it forms a very insoluble compound.

Test.—Calcium chloride gives a white precipitate, insoluble in acetic, but soluble in hydrochloric acid.

PYROGALLIC ACID sublimes as white, feathery crystals when gallic acid is heated. Used in gas analysis to absorb oxygen, as a deoxidizer in photography, and as a hair dye.

Test.—A blue color with ferrous, and a red with ferric salts.

SALICYLIC ACID.—Formerly prepared from salicin, but now made by a patented process from carbolic acid. A very pure acid may be obtained from oil of wintergreen, which consists mainly of methyl salicylate. This, treated with potassium hydrate, forms methyl hydrate (methyl alcohol) and potassium salicylate; and if to this hydrochloric acid be added, potassium chloride will be formed, and salicylic acid will fall in a mass of silky, white crystals. Salicylic acid is scarcely soluble in cold water, hence the salicylate of sodium is usually prescribed, which is not only more soluble, but less irritating to mucous membranes.

Test.—Intense violet with a ferric salt.

SUCCINIC ACID was first obtained from amber (*succinum*), but is now made by fermenting malic acid.

TANNIC ACID, OR TANNIN.—This is the active principle of the vegetable astringents; usually obtained from oak galls; a greenish or brownish powder, very soluble in water, of a rough, astringent taste. It precipitates solutions of salts of the alkaloids and most metals. It precipitates gelatin and other albuminoid substances, a fact that explains the process of tanning raw hides. With ferric solutions tannin gives a black precipitate (black ink).

TARTARIC ACID—$H_2C_4H_4O_6$, or H_2T.—Tartrates exist in the juices of many fruits. Grape juice contains much acid tartrate of potassium (KHT), which, being very insoluble in an alcoholic menstruum, is precipitated on the sides of the cask whenever the wine ferments. This forms *argol*, the principal source of cream of tartar and tartaric acid. Tartaric acid forms colorless crystals, very soluble, and of a sharp, agreeable, sour taste.

VALERIANIC ACID—$HC_5H_9O_2$.—This substance was first obtained from valerian root; but now it is made artificially by oxidizing amylic alcohol by means of sulphuric acid and potassium bichromate.

Valerianic acid is a colorless liquid, possessing the disagreeable odor of valerian.

The Carbohydrates.—These substances are closely related to the alcohols, and by some classed as such. They are so named because they contain carbon (six or twelve atoms), and the hydrogen and oxygen they contain are in the exact proportion to form water. They constitute the bulk of plants. They are divided into three groups:—

1. AMYLOSES ($C_6H_{10}O_5$), which include cellulin, starch, dextrin, glycogen, gums, etc.
2. SACCHAROSES ($C_{12}H_{22}O_{11}$), including cane sugar, milk sugar, etc.
3. GLUCOSES ($C_6H_{12}O_6$), such as grape sugar (glucose), fruit sugar, etc.

Although the members of each of these groups differ widely in their physical and chemical properties, still they consist of the same elements in exactly the same proportions and have the same formula. Such bodies are said to be *isomeric*.

AMYLOSES—($C_6H_{10}O_5$).—CELLULIN—*Cellulose, Lignin*—forms the cell-walls and tissues of plants. Woody fibre, cotton, linen, and unsized paper are almost pure cellulin. Dissolves in a solution of cupric oxide in ammonia. Acids precipitate it as a white mass, which, mixed with camphor and compressed, is *celluloid*. Unsized paper dipped into moderately strong sulphuric acid, washed and dried, has its fibres agglutinated, loses its porosity, becomes very tough, and is sold as *artificial parchment* for dialysers, diplomas, etc.

Nitro-cellulose, or *Gun Cotton*, a powerful explosive, is cotton that has been dipped into a mixture of nitric and sulphuric acids, and then washed and dried. Its solution in ether is *collodion*. The *flexible* collodion contains a little turpentine and castor oil; the *styptic* collodion contains twenty per cent. tannin.

STARCH—*Amylum*—the most important member of the carbohydrates, and a valuable food; found in the roots, stems and seeds of all plants. Starch is a white powder, consisting of granules, formed of concentric layers, like an onion. These granules have all a similar appearance. Yet those from different kinds of plants differ enough to enable one, by microscopic examination, to determine the source of any starch (Fig. 39).

When starch is boiled the granules swell and burst, casting the

PART II.—ORGANIC CHEMISTRY. 113

starch into the water, forming mucilage of starch, which is used for laundrying and for surgical dressings. Starch is a very valuable food. The best test for starch is iodine, with which it forms a blue. Heat discharges the blue, but it returns on cooling.

DEXTRIN—*British Gum*—is the gum used on postage stamps, etc. It may be made from starch in various ways, one of which is by heating it to 300° F. It is very soluble, and gives no blue with iodine.

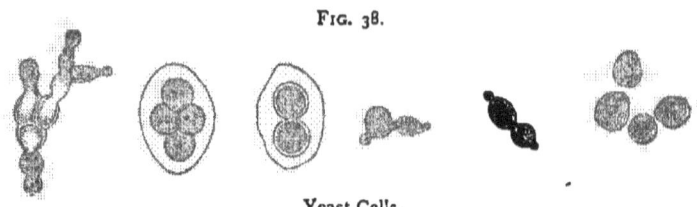

FIG. 38.

Yeast Cells.

GLYCOGEN—(*Generator of Glucose*)—is found in the animal economy, especially in the liver. Like dextrin, it is a derivative of starch, but differs from it in being soluble, and giving only a wine-

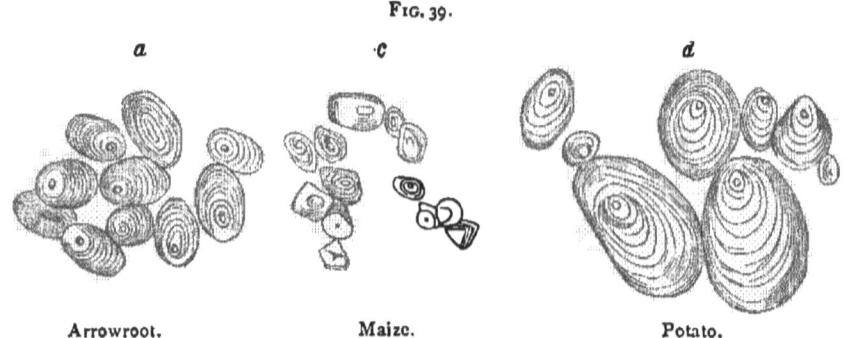

FIG. 39.

a   c   d

Arrowroot.   Maize.   Potato.

color with iodine. It seems to be the form in which the carbohydrates are stored up, to be used by the system as necessity arises.

GUMS are a class of substances soluble in water, but insoluble in alcohol. A type of the class is *gum Arabic*.

SACCHAROSES—$C_{12}H_{22}O_{11}$.—CANE SUGAR—*Beet Sugar, Sucrose.* Very abundant in the sugar-cane, sugar-maple, beet-root, etc. It is the most soluble, perfectly crystallizable, and sweetest of the sugars, and the one most used for domestic purposes. Its aqueous solution is called *simple syrup* (*syrupus simplex*).

MILK SUGAR, as its name implies, occurs in milk; harder, less soluble, and less sweet than cane-sugar. Used in the trituration of medicines.

GLUCOSES—$C_6H_{12}O_6$.—GLUCOSE—*Grape Sugar, Diabetic Sugar.*—Found associated with other sugars in most plants, especially in the grape; but the source of most interest to the physician is the animal economy. This is the sugar of diabetic urine, and the ability to detect it with ease and certainty in such conditions is a necessity to the practitioner of the present day.

Glucose is not so sweet nor so soluble and crystallizable as cane-sugar. Having great affinity for oxygen it is a valuable reducing agent, and on this property most of its tests depend. Boiled with a dilute mineral acid or allowed to remain under the influence of certain animal and vegetable ferments,* warm and moist, the amyloses and

---

* FERMENTS.—These are certain nitrogenous bodies, animal and vegetable, which by some means not clearly understood cause many organic compounds to decompose with the production of other and simpler substances, the ferments themselves being unaffected. Ferments are of two classes:—
1. The *unorganized*, or *soluble* ferments. Among these are: (*a*) *Diastase*, or *maltin*, formed from the gluten and serving to convert the starch of the seed into glucose. Malt, which is sprouted barley, contains it in abundance, and is used to convert meal (starch) into glucose for fermentation in the manufacture of alcoholic liquors, and in medicine as a digestive agent. The ptyalin of saliva and a pancreatic ferment act like diastase. (*b*) *Pepsin*, of the gastric juice, and (*c*) *Trypsin*, of the pancreatic fluid, both of which serve to convert the albuminoids into peptones; the one in acid, and the other in alkaline solution.
2. *Organized Ferments.*—When their spores are carried by the atmosphere or otherwise into a suitable, fermentable liquid, and kept warm (68° to 105° F.), these ferments grow and proliferate with great rapidity, inducing fermentative changes in a few hours. The most important of these ferments are: (*a*) Yeast (*torula cerevisiæ*), shown in Fig. 38. This converts glucose into alcohol and carbon dioxide (vinous fermentation). (*b*) *Acetic acid ferment* (*mycoderma aceti*), commonly called "mother of vinegar," grows on solutions containing alcohol, which it helps to oxidize into acetic acid. (*c*) *Thrush fungus* (*oïdium albicans*) grows within the mouths of ill-kept children. It induces a slight alcoholic fermentation. (*d*) *Lactic* and *Butyric* ferments go together, the one preceding and the other closely following. These fermentations occur in intestinal indigestion, and the gas evolved produces flatulent colic.

Putrefaction (the spontaneous decomposition of nitrogenous organized bodies) is accompanied, if not caused, by microörganisms, usually bacteria. *Decay*, on the other hand, is the gradual decomposition of organic bodies by the slow action of oxygen, and does not depend on living organisms.

saccharoses are converted into glucose. The reaction consists in the addition of H_2O to the molecule, thus:—

Starch. Water. Glucose. Cane Sugar. Water. Glucose.
$C_6H_{10}O_5 + H_2O = C_6H_{12}O_6.$ $C_{12}H_{22}O_{11} + H_2O = 2C_6H_{12}O_6.$

When starch and cane-sugar are eaten the digestive ferments (pancreatin and ptyalin) convert them into glucose. The ferment (diastase), developed in a germinating seed, converts the starch into glucose, which is readily assimilated by the sprouting plant.

Glucose is so easily made by boiling cellulin, but more especially starches, with sulphuric acid, that it has become a common adulterant or substitute for cane-sugar, especially syrup. This would be harmless but for the fact that the cheap acid used is apt to be contaminated with lead, arsenic, etc.

Glucosides.—This class includes a numerous class of neutral substances, mostly of vegetable origin, which, though differing greatly among themselves, possess one common property, viz.: When acted upon by a ferment or a dilute acid, they decompose, producing among other things, glucose. Their chemical constitution is not thoroughly understood, but probably they are ethers of glucose. They generally have marked physiological action, and are therefore the active principles of the drugs in which they occur. Their names generally allude to their origin and terminate with "*-in.*" A few of the most important are:—

Amygdalin, exists in the bitter almond (amygdala), in the leaves of cherry laurel, and in the seeds of peaches, cherries and plums, associated with an albuminoid ferment, *emulsin* or *synaptase*, which in the presence of heat and moisture decomposes the amygdalin into hydrocyanic acid, benzaldehyde and glucose.

Salicin is the bitter principle in the bark of the willow (*salix*). It has been employed as a substitute and adulterant of quinine, from which it may be known by the blood red it gives with sulphuric acid.

Tannin, or *Tannic Acid*, is also a glucoside. This explains why certain fruits, *e. g.*, persimmons, on ripening, lose their rough, astringent taste and get sweet.

Myronic Acid exists in black mustard, associated with an albuminous ferment, capable of converting it into glucose and another substance (allyl sulphocyanate) to which the virtue of mustard is due.

Hot water, by coagulating this ferment, renders a mustard plaster inert.

Indican occurs in various plants, the *indigofera ;* also in urine, being derived from indol, a weak base produced by the pancreas and taken up from the alimentary canal.* It is a brownish, bitter, syrupy liquid, which, when fermented or treated with dilute acid, forms indigo-blue and a kind of glucose.

Other important glucosides are: *Arbutin, cathartic acid, colocynthin, digitalin, elaterin, gentianin, glycyrrhizin* (licorice), *jalapin, santonin, saponin, solanin,* etc.

Nitrogenous Bodies.—To the physician these are of extreme interest, for to this class belong most of the tissues and waste products of the body and of our most potent remedies and virulent poisons.

PROTEIDS—*Albumin, Globulin, Vitellin, Casein, Fibrin, Peptones, Gelatin, Chondrin, etc.*—These substances, formed in plants and appropriated by animals, constitute the greater part of the solid portion of the fluids and tissues of the body, and play the chief part in physiological processes. Their molecular constitution (rational formula) is not definitely known, but their composition seems to be $C_{72}H_{112}N_{18}S$. They are amorphous, colloid (not crystalline) and, except peptones, are not osmotic (do not diffuse through animal membranes). When dry, they are easily preserved, but when moist, prone to putrefy. They are rendered insoluble by various substances, by which means they are often recognized.

Tests.—(1) They are all precipitated by alcohol in excess and in time coagulated. (2) Heated with strong nitric acid they turn *yellow,* and on the addition of an alkali (ammonia, soda or potash) become *orange.*

BODIES OF THE AMMONIA TYPE.—Taking the molecule of ammonia, NH_3, as a basis, and by substituting for one or more atoms of its hydrogen one or more organic radicals, or combinations of radicals, we can obtain a large number of interesting and important substances. Many of these substances have trade names in allusion to some use or property, or in abbreviation of their chemical names. In chemistry they bear the names of the radicals entering into their composition, and end in "*-amine*" when those radicals are electro-positive, or in "*-amide*" when electro-negative. For example:—

Amines—

Ammonia. Ethylamine. Phenylamine. Trimethylamine.

$N \begin{cases} H \\ H \\ H \end{cases}$; $N \begin{cases} C_2H_5 \text{ (ethyl)} \\ H \\ H \end{cases}$; $N \begin{cases} C_6H_5 \text{ (phenyl)} \\ H \\ H \end{cases}$; $N \begin{cases} CH_3 \text{ (methyl)} \\ CH_3 \text{ "} \\ CH_3 \text{ "} \end{cases}$ etc.

Like ammonia, these bodies are alkaline and combine with acids to form salts, appropriating instead of displacing their hydrogen, *e. g.* $NH_3 + HCl = NH_4Cl$, ammonium chloride or ammonia hydrochloride; in like manner $NH_2(C_2H_5) + HCl = NH_2(C_2H_5)HCl$, ethylamine hydrochloride.

Amides—

Ammonia (Amine). Acetamide. Acetanilide (Phenyl Acetamide). Carbamide (Urea).

$N \begin{cases} H \\ H \\ H \end{cases}$; $N \begin{cases} H \\ H \\ C_2H_3O \text{ (acetic rad.)} \end{cases}$; $N \begin{cases} H \\ C_2H_3O \\ C_6H_5 \text{ (phenyl)} \end{cases}$; $N \begin{cases} H \\ H \\ \end{cases} > CO$ $N \begin{cases} H \\ H \end{cases}$

Aniline (Phenylamine) is a colorless liquid, but its compounds (the aniline dyes) are coloring matters of great brilliancy.*
$N \begin{cases} C_6H_5 \\ H \\ H \end{cases}$ They are sometimes contaminated with arsenic used in their manufacture.

Trimethylamine is sometimes confounded with propylamine. It
$N \begin{cases} CH_3 \\ CH_3 \\ CH_3 \end{cases}$ is a colorless, volatile alkaloid, with an ammoniacal, fishy odor. It is found in many animal and vegetable substances, but obtained from pickled herring. The hydrochloride is the salt used. Dose, ten to fifteen grains.

Antifebrin (acetanilide). This is a derivative of aniline in which
$N \begin{cases} C_6H_5 \\ H \\ C_2H_3O_2 \end{cases}$ the acetic radical is made to displace an atom of hydrogen. A crystalline, odorless, solid, slightly soluble in warm water, very soluble in alcohol. In doses of five to ten grains, repeated every two or three hours, it is an antipyretic and sedative. It is said not to affect the healthy temperature, but to rapidly lower a fever.

*****Experiment.**—Dissolve a few drops of aniline in water in two test-tubes. To one add solution of chlorinated lime—a purple color is produced; to the other add some sulphuric acid and potassium chromate mixture—a blue color appears.

Phenacetine. The formula shows that this substance is closely
allied to acetanilide. A white crystalline
powder, but slightly soluble in water. In
doses of fifteen grains it causes a fall of temperature and a profuse sweat. Its effect is more persistent, and perhaps more dangerous than antipyrin, producing symptoms of aniline poisoning with hæmoglobinuria and jaundice.

$$N \begin{cases} C_6H_4-O-C_2H_5 \\ H \\ C_2H_3O \end{cases}$$

Antipyrine, $C_{11}H_{12}N_2O$, a derivative of the artificial alkaloid, chinoline, is a white crystalline powder, soluble in water and alcohol, of a slight tarry taste and odor. With nitrous acid it forms a poisonous precipitate, and is therefore incompatible with spirits of nitrous ether. The hydrochloride is the salt used. In doses of ten to fifteen grains it is a valuable antipyretic and anodyne.

Alkaloids (alkali-like).—These bodies are mostly of vegetable origin and bear a close analogy to the preceding, for they are ammonia substitution compounds, alkaline in reaction, and combine with acids to form salts. Of late years chemists have made substances very similar to, if not identical with, some of the natural alkaloids; and the time seems not far distant when our most costly alkaloids will be made cheaply by artificial means. In plants alkaloids are not found free, but combined with some vegetable acid forming a salt. Their salts (except tannates) are usually soluble and intensely bitter; the free alkaloids being much less soluble, are much less bitter. Those alkaloids (as conine and nicotine) that contain no oxygen are liquid; but the great majority of them are white powders.

Alkaloids are so seldom prescribed in the free state that when the simple name of an alkaloid is written in a prescription the druggist puts up its most common salt. The names of alkaloids end in "*-ine,*" and are derived from the names of the plants in which they exist or from some characteristic property.

The intense effect alkaloids exert on the animal organism makes them generally the active principles of the drugs in which they are found. But the active principle of a drug is not always an alkaloid. The alkaloids include the majority of our most potent remedies and powerful poisons. Tannin is a common antidote, but most important is the prompt evacuation of the stomach and the intelligent use of physiological antagonists.

The alkaloids, even those of medical interest, are so numerous that

PART II.—ORGANIC CHEMISTRY.   119

to give each separate consideration would cover a great portion of the materia medica. We can mention but a few of the most important.

NAME.	FORMULA.	SOURCE.	REMARKS.
Morphine	$C_{17}H_{19}NO_3$	Opium	Crystalline; morphia gives a blue with Fe_2Cl_6, and a red with HNO_3. These alkaloids and several others exist in opium in combination with meconic acid, which gives with Fe_2Cl_6 a red color not discharged by $HgCl_2$.
Codeine	$C_{18}H_{21}NO_3$	"	
Narcotine	$C_{22}H_{23}NO_7$	"	
Narceine	$C_{23}H_{29}NO_9$	"	
Apomorphine	$C_{17}H_{17}NO_2$	Morphine	Made by heating morphine with HCl; a systemic emetic.
Quinine	$C_{20}H_{24}N_2O_2$	Cinchona bark	All crystalline except quinoidine, which is a resinous mass. To test for quinine, add chlorine water, shake, and then add aq. ammonia; a green color.
Quinidine	"		
Quinicine	"		
Quinoidine	"		
Cinchonine	$C_{20}H_{24}N_2O$		
Cinchonidine	"		
Cinchonicine	"		
Strychnine	$C_{21}H_{22}N_2O_2$	Nux vomica	Crystals; gives a purple with H_2SO_4 and $K_2Cr_2O_7$.
Brucine	$C_{23}H_{26}N_2O_4$	"	Crystals; gives a red with HNO_3.
Aconitine	$C_{30}H_{47}NO_7$	Aconite	Crystals; very poisonous.
Colchicine	$C_{17}H_{19}NO_5$	Colchicum	
Veratrine	$C_{32}H_{52}N_2O_8$	Veratrum	
Atropine	$C_{17}H_{23}NO_3$	Belladonna	Crystals; used to dilate the pupils.
Hyoscyamine	$C_{15}H_{23}NO_3$	Hyoscyamus	
Homatropine	$C_{16}H_{22}NO_3$	Atropine	
Caffeine		Coffee	Crystals; soluble in water; weakly basic.
Theine		Tea	Crystals; soluble in water; weakly basic; anodyne.
Cocaine		Coco leaves	Crystals; soluble in water; weakly basic; local anæsthetic.
Physostigmine (Eserine)	$C_{15}H_{21}N_3O_2$	Physostigma (Calabar bean)	Crystals; contracts the pupils.
Pilocarpine	$C_{11}H_{16}N_2O_2$	Jaborandi	Crystals; a powerful diaphoretic.
Urea	CH_4N_2O	Urine	Crystals; may be made artificially by heating NH_4CNO.
Nicotine	C_5H_7N	Tobacco	Liquid; powerful poison.
Conine	$C_8H_{15}N$	Hemlock	" " "

PROMAÏNES (πτῶμα, a corpse).—This name is given to certain alkaloids or amines formed in animal and some vegetable bodies during putrefaction, and in some pathological conditions during life. These are the products of bacteria, each species producing its own peculiar ptomaïne. Thus, the typhoid-bacillus produces typhotoxine; the tetanus-bacillus, tetanine, etc. Many think the symptoms of the specific fevers are only the effects of the ptomaïnes so produced, for the characteristic symptoms of the disease may be produced by the administration of its ptomaïne. The poisoning that frequently results from eating spoiled meat, fish, etc., is due to ptomaïnes. The symptoms resemble those of the vegetable alkaloids, except that there is usually more gastro-intestinal irritation. The fact that certain ptomaïnes give physiological effects and chemical tests like such alkaloids as strychnine, morphine, conine, nicotine, atropine and veratrine, is apt to, and doubtless has often, caused the condemnation of the innocent.

Among the non-poisonous ptomaïnes may be mentioned *putrescine*, *cadaverine* and *neuridine*. Among the poisonous are: *choline*, which acts like curarine; *muscarine*, from poisonous mushroons (muscarius); *tetanine*, *tetanotoxine* and *spasmotoxine*, produced by the tetanus-bacillus and causing (?) the symptoms of tetanus; *typhotoxine*, produced by the typhoid-bacillus and causing (?) the symptoms of typhoid fever, and *tyrotoxine*, found by Dr. Vaughan in poisonous cheese and milk and causing the symptoms of cholera infantum.

LEUCOMAÏNES are a class of alkaloidal substances produced in the *living* body as the result of fermentative changes or of the processes of retrograde metamorphosis, and are closely related to urea and uric acid. They are eliminated in the various excreta, the urine, fæces, perspiration, etc. If retained, as in uræmia, or produced in abnormal amounts, as in dyspepsia, they act deleteriously on the nerve centres causing vertigo, lassitude, drowsiness, vomiting, purging and coma. Some elevate while others lower the temperature. Of the more important we may mention creatine, creatinine and xanthine.

The chemistry of the ptomaïnes and leucomaïnes is new and still incomplete.

PART III.

THE URINE.

The urine is a fluid secreted continuously by the kidneys, and is the chief means by which the nitrogenous waste of the body is discharged.* A specimen, to be representative, should be a portion of the whole twenty-fours' urine, for considerable variation in composition and properties may occur during the day. Especially is this true of traces of albumin and sugar. When this is impracticable, that passed before breakfast is generally preferable, because farthest from a meal. When significant variations during the day are suspected, several specimens may be taken at different hours. For *microscopical examination* a few ounces of the urine in a stoppered vial, or better still, in a covered conical glass (Fig. 40) are set aside for several hours until the sediment has settled to the bottom and can be examined.

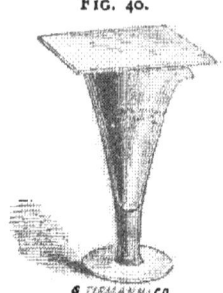

FIG. 40.

---

* The rationale of its secretion is one of transudation, osmosis, and cell elaboration. Owing to the resistance encountered by the blood in its exit through the efferent vessel, there is an increase of blood-pressure in the Malpighian tuft and a transudation of the water of the blood with some dissolved salts into the capsule. From loss of water the blood is very much thickened when it reaches the second capillary system surrounding the convoluted tubes, which contain the thin, watery transudation from the Malpighian bodies. Here are the essential elements of a complete osmometer—an animal membrane, composed of the thin wall of the capillary and the delicate basement membrane of the tube, with a dense fluid (the thickened blood) on one side and a thin saline solution on the other. An interchange now takes place of the water from the tube to the blood, and of the products of retrograde metamorphosis (urea, etc.), and salts from the blood to the tubes, concentrating the fluid in the latter, making it urine, while the albuminous constituents of the blood, not being osmotic, are retained. An elaborative function has long been

Physical Properties.—Normal urine is a *transparent, aqueous fluid, of a pale yellow color, characteristic odor, acid reaction, and a specific gravity of* 1020 *when passed in the average quantity of about forty-five fluid ounces in the twenty-four hours.* This description is to be taken with much allowance, for very wide variations occur even in health. With these variations the student must become thoroughly familiar before he is capable of interpreting a specimen. Therefore the physical properties will be considered more particularly.

Quantity.—*In health* this depends upon (*a*) the amount of water ingested, and (*b*) its vicarious elimination by the skin, lungs, and bowels. *Pathologically* it is increased in diabetes, also in hysterical conditions associated with convulsions and high arterial pressure, and after the administration of diuretics.

Transparency.—Normal urine is not always transparent, nor is transparent always normal. Some degree of opacity may be due to: (*a*) *Mucus*, with some entangled epithelial cells, which may be observed in many specimens of healthy urine, especially of females, because of the larger area of mucous surface in that sex. (*b*) *Urates* (of Na, K, Ca, and Mg), which often form a precipitate in urine, especially when allowed to stand over night in a cold room. The test for this sediment is heat, which quickly dissipates it. (*c*) *Earthy phosphates* (of Ca and Mg), which may give an opacity to normal urine, especially if it is alkaline or even weakly acid. The test for this sediment is the addition of a few drops of any acid which promptly clears it up, while heat would only increase it. (*d*) *Fungi* (bacteria, penicillia, sarcinæ, etc.), especially in decomposing urine.

A urine may be abnormally opaque from the above causes, or from the presence of blood or pus. When due to blood or pus the opacity is increased by heat or acids because of the precipitation of albumin always present in *liquor sanguinis* and *liquor puris*.

Fluidity.—Healthy urine is never otherwise than an aqueous fluid,

---

attributed to the epithelial cells lining the convoluted tubes, for it was observed that whenever the tubes lost their epithelial lining (as in some forms of Bright's disease), urea, etc., failed to be eliminated. This function of the cells may be demonstrated by injecting into the veins of a rabbit a solution of sulph-indigotate of sodium. If the animal be killed within a few minutes, none of the coloring matter will be found in the capsules, while the cells lining the tubes will be stained blue. If, however, an hour be allowed to elapse, even the cells will be found colorless and the coloring matter will be seen only in the urine.

flowing and dripping with ease; but in certain diseased conditions, abnormal quantities of mucus, or the presence of pus or fat, especially if the urine be allowed to decompose and become very alkaline, may give rise to viscidity.

Color.—*Healthy* variations in color depend mainly upon the amount of water and the consequent degree of concentration or dilution of the solid constituents. Aside from abnormal degrees of the above, *pathological* variations in color may be the result of (*a*) an increase or diminution of the normal coloring matters, as in fevers, etc.; (*b*) the presence of abnormal substances, as biliary and blood coloring matters. Moreover, the urine may be colored after the administration of certain drugs, as senna, santonin, rhubarb, prickly pear, etc.

Odor.—When freshly passed, urine has, in addition to its characteristic odor, an aromatic fragrance due to certain volatile ethers. Alkaline urine has an ammoniacal odor, unless the alkalinity be due to fixed alkali, when the smell is fainty and sickening, like that of horses' urine. Diabetic urine exhales a sweetish smell. In certain forms of dyspepsia and liver trouble, the odor of the urine is almost pathognomonic. Medicines and certain articles of food often impart a peculiar odor, as turpentine the odor of violets, and asparagus and cauliflower a rank, disgusting smell.

Reaction.—Normally the urine of the whole twenty-four hours will average an acid reaction; but great variations occur during the day. Before meals it will have a high degree of acidity, but after eating becomes nearly neutral, or even alkaline. This is due to the ingestion of food which is largely alkaline and to the abstraction of acidulous principles from the blood to form acid gastric juice. It has also been observed that urine passed on rising in the morning is especially acid. This is probably due to the fact that during sleep less carbonic acid is exhaled from the lungs and less perspiration (acid) given off by the skin. The reaction of the urine is important to the physician, as it may favor or prevent the formation of sediments and concretions or irritation of the kidneys and bladder. The acidity of urine is due, not to free acid, but to acid sodium phosphate (NaH_2PO_4) occurring in consequence of carbonic, uric, and hippuric acids, seizing on to a portion of the sodium of the basic phosphate.

An *acid fermentation*, attended with decomposition of mucus and coloring matters and a production of acetic and lactic acids, sometimes occurs in urine that has stood for some time at a moderate temperature. After a while, more quickly in warm weather, the *alkaline fermentation* begins, caused by the development of the micrococcus

FIG. 41.

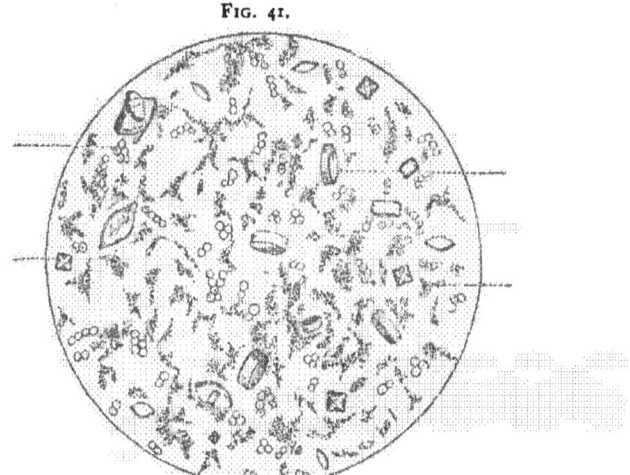

Acid Fermentation.

FIG. 42.

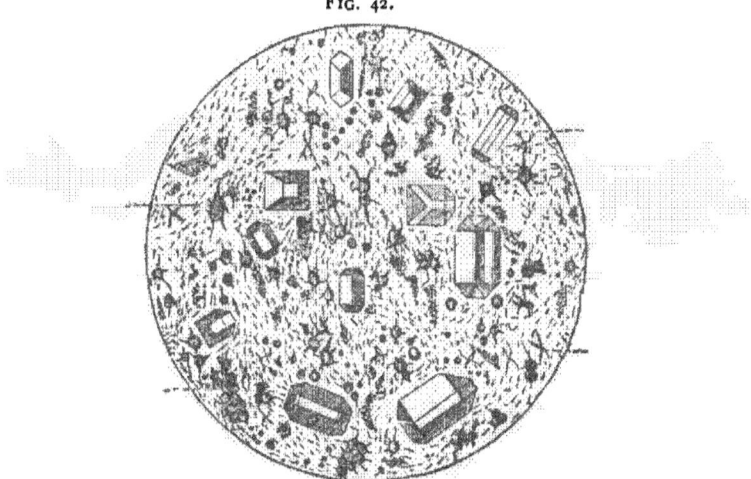

Alkaline Fermentation.

ureæ (Pasteur). The urea is converted into ammonium carbonate, thus :—

$$CH_4N_2O + 2H_2O = (NH_4)_2CO_3.$$

This gives the urine an ammoniacal odor and alkaline reaction, and it becomes opaque from the precipitation of urate of ammonium and the earthy phosphates and the development of bacteria. Pus and blood, or vessels tainted with urine previously fermented, greatly hasten this change.

The reaction is determined by litmus paper. If acid, the blue litmus is turned red; if alkaline, the red litmus is turned blue; if neutral, there is no change in either. If alkalinity be due to ammonia (volatile alkali), the blued paper gets red again on drying.

Specific Gravity.—Though the average specific gravity is 1020, it exhibits, even in health, great variations, the extremes being 1002 after copious use of water and diuretics, and 1040 after abstinence from fluid and the elimination of water through other means, as profuse perspiration or copious diarrhœa. The amount of solids varying but little in health, fluctuations in specific gravity are due mainly to variations in the amount of water, and, as long as the inverse proportion between specific gravity and volume of urine is preserved, variations need cause no alarm.

Specific gravity is usually measured by an instrument called a hydrometer or *urinometer* (Fig. 43), which is a hollow glass float, weighted with mercury and having a long, graduated neck. The graduation begins above at 1000, because the heavier the urine the less deeply will the instrument sink and the further the neck will protrude from the surface. It is well to test a new urinometer by immersing it in water at 60° F. (15.5° C.), into which it should sink to 0 or 1000 on the scale. Urinometers are usually provided with a cylinder or jar, as shown in the figure, but a large test-tube will answer. This is about three-fourths filled; the urinometer is then introduced, and when still, the specific gravity is read off. The cylinder or test-tube should not be too narrow, lest the urinometer be attracted to and catch against the sides, and not rise as high or sink as low as it should. The fluid being attracted up around the stem, the reading should be made not along the line $c\,d$, as in the diagram, suggested by Dr. Leffmann, of Philadelphia, but $a\,b$,

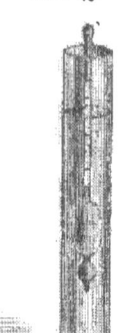

FIG. 43.

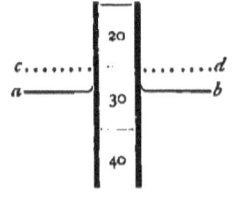

which represents the true level of the liquid. To approximate the amount of solids in any urine: (*a*) The last two figures of the specific gravity represent the number of grains of solids to the fluid ounce; (*b*) doubling the last two figures of the specific gravity, gives the per cent. Thus, if a urine be of specific gravity 1020, and the daily volume fifty ounces, (*a*) 20 (grains per fluid ounce), multiplied by 50 (ounces daily volume) gives 1000 grains of solids per diem; (*b*) .020 $\times$ 2 = .040 or 4 per cent., which multiplied by 50 (ounces daily volume) gives 2 ounces of solids per diem.

CHEMICAL CONSTITUENTS.—The average composition of a thousand parts of urine is about as follows:—

Organic.	Water,	950.00
	Urea,	26.20
	Kreatine and kreatinine,	.80
	Urates of sodium and potassium,	1.45
	Hippurates of sodium and potassium,	.70
	Mucus and coloring matters,	.35
Inorganic.	Phosphates of sodium and potassium,	3.75
	Phosphates of calcium and magnesium,	.90
	Chlorides of sodium and potassium,	12.55
	Sulphates of sodium and potassium,	3.30
		1000.00

Pathologically there may be present also albumin, glucose, blood, bile, etc., besides various sediments.

UREA—CH_4N_2O.—This is the most constant and abundant organic constituent of the urine, and, being the main nitrogenous excretion, it is the index of nitrogenous waste, whether of food or tissue. Its average amount is about one ounce *per diem*.

Urea may be obtained by extracting it from the urine, or artificially by heating cyanate of ammonium with which it is isomeric (NH_4-CNO = CH_4N_2O).

It crystallizes in colorless prisms, very soluble in water, and behaves like an alkaloid, combining readily with nitric and oxalic acids to form salts. Both of these salts may, by adding nitric or oxalic acid, be precipitated from concentrated urine as colorless, rhombic or hexagonal plates. (Fig. 44, *c*.)

In the course of many diseases it is important to estimate the amount of urea excreted day by day. A rough estimate may be based on the specific gravity. For, since urea is the largest solid ingredient in urine, it follows that if sugar be absent, albumin in small amount or removed, and the amount of chlorides normal, variations in specific gravity must be due mainly to variations in amount of urea.

The exact methods most generally employed consist in decomposing the urine into nitrogen and carbon dioxide, by means of sodium hypochlorite or hypobromite, and measuring either the volume of gas evolved or the specific gravity lost by the decomposition.

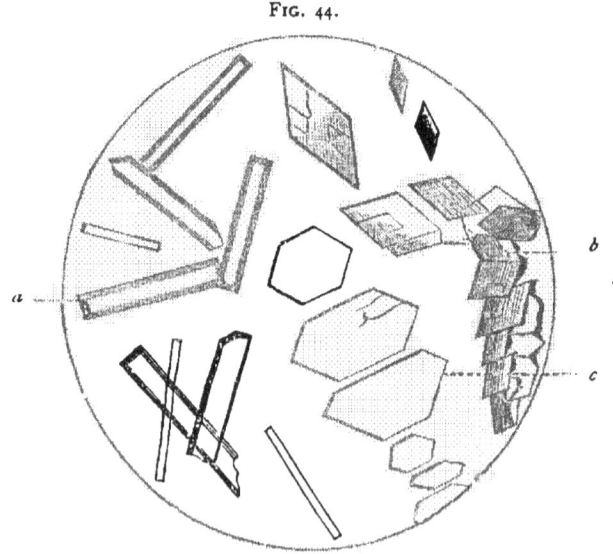

FIG. 44.

(*a*) Urea; (*b*) hexagonal plates; and (*c*) smaller scales, or rhombic plates of Urea Nitrate.

Davy's Hypochlorite Method.—A graduated tube closed at one end is one-third filled with mercury. A measured quantity of the urine (a drachm or half drachm, according to capacity of tube) is then added, and the tube is next filled to the brim with the hypochlorite solution (liq. sod. chloratæ, U. S. P.). Closing the opening with the thumb, the tube is inverted over a strong solution of common salt in a dish. (Fig. 45.) The mercury runs out and the salt water rises to take its place, while the urine and soda mixture, being lighter, remain in the upper part of the tube. Here the gas from the decomposing urea collects. The decomposition is complete in three or four hours, when the amount of the gas may be read off by the graduations upon the tube, every cubic inch representing .64 grain (or 1 cubic centimetre representing 2.5 milligrams) of urea.

Doremus' Hypobromite Method.—The sodium hypobromite is prepared by adding 1 cubic centimetre of bromine to 10 cubic centimetres of sodium hydrate solution (100 grammes to 250 cubic centimetres of water, or 6 ounces to 1 pint) and diluting with 10 cubic centimetres of water. Tilt the ureometer (Fig. 46), and pour the hypobromite into the long arm, completely filling it. Draw the urine to be tested into

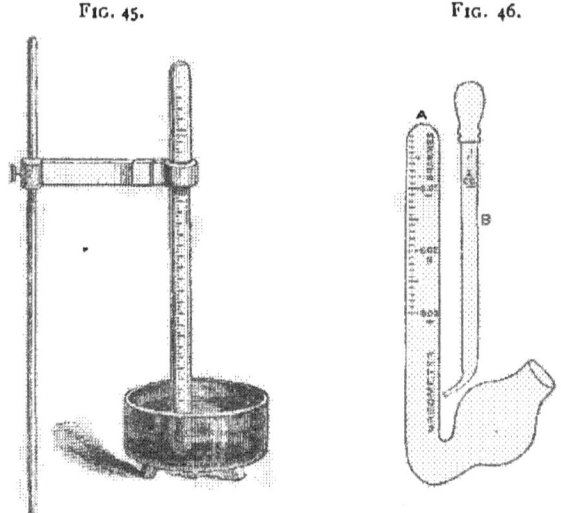

FIG. 45.   FIG. 46.

the pipette to the graduation. Pass the pipette into the ureometer as far as the bend, and compress the nipple slowly. The urine will rise through the hypobromite, and the gas evolved will collect in the upper part of the tube. The ureometer is graduated to indicate either the number of milligrammes of urea to the cubic centimetre of urine or the number of grains to the fluidounce.

Fowler's Method.—The specific gravity of the urine is carefully determined as well as that of the liq. sodæ chloratæ (U. S. P.) to be used. One volume of the urine is mixed with exactly seven volumes of the liq. sod. chlor. and set aside for two hours, or until effervescence ceases. The specific gravity is again taken. As the reaction begins immediately on mixing the fluids, the specific gravity of the mixture must be calculated. This is done by adding to the specific gravity of the urine seven times that of the liq. sod. chlor. and dividing the sum by eight. Each degree of difference in specific gravity of the mixture before and after the decomposition represents three and a half grains of urea to the fluidounce of the day's urine.

Example:—

	Ounces.
Quantity of urine in twenty-four hours,	46
Sp. gr. of the urine,	1020
Sp. gr. liq. sod. chloratæ,	1042
(Calculated) Sp. gr. mixture ($\frac{1042 \times 7 + 1020}{8} =$),	1039.2 +
(Actual) Sp. gr. mixture after reaction,	1036.2

$1039.2 - 1036.2 = 3$; $3 \times 3\frac{1}{2} = 10\frac{1}{2}$ grs. of urea to the ounce of urine; $10\frac{1}{2} \times 46 = 483$ grs. of urea passed in twenty-four hours.

KREATINE AND KREATININE, substances closely allied to urea, exist in urine in such small amounts as to be of no practical significance, and need only to be mentioned in this connection.

URIC ACID is found in the urine of carnivora: in that of herbivora it is largely replaced by an analogous substance—hippuric acid (Fig. 55). Gout is characterized by an increased production of uric acid, and the so-called "chalk-stone" deposit in joints during that disease is sodium urate. Free uric acid is so very insoluble that whenever it exists in urine it is always a precipitate. It appears as minute reddish grains, which under the microscope are seen to be modifications of rhombic crystals, always stained with the coloring matter of the urine. They often deviate widely from the typical rhomb, as shown in Figs. 47 and 48, but an experienced eye will readily recognize them. Normally, uric acid, as soon as formed, unites with the alkaline bases to form *urates.* They are very soluble in warm water, but more sparingly so in cold. Therefore a urine, though clear when freshly passed and warm, may exhibit a copious precipitate upon becoming cold, as on a winter night. This precipitate is easily recognized by its dissolving upon warming. Urates of **sodium and magnesium** generally appear under the microscope as **amorphous powders** in moss-like aggregations, but occasionally as bundles of small needles, as shown in Fig. 49. The urate of ammonium, a result of the alkaline fermentation, occurs as **opaque, brown spherules,** smooth or with spiculæ like a thorn-apple (Fig. 42). The acid urates are less soluble than the normal, and often precipitate when the urine is very acid or when an acid is added, as in the nitric-acid test for albumin.

The *murexid test* for uric acid and the urates is one of great beauty. Place some of the sediment in a porcelain dish, add a drop or two of nitric acid, and carefully evaporate almost to dryness. If a few drops of ammonia be added, it assumes a beautiful purple color.

If uric acid be present, a beautiful purple color will appear whenever a few drops of ammonia are added; or better still (Earp), if the dish be inverted over another in which a dry ammonium salt is volatilized.

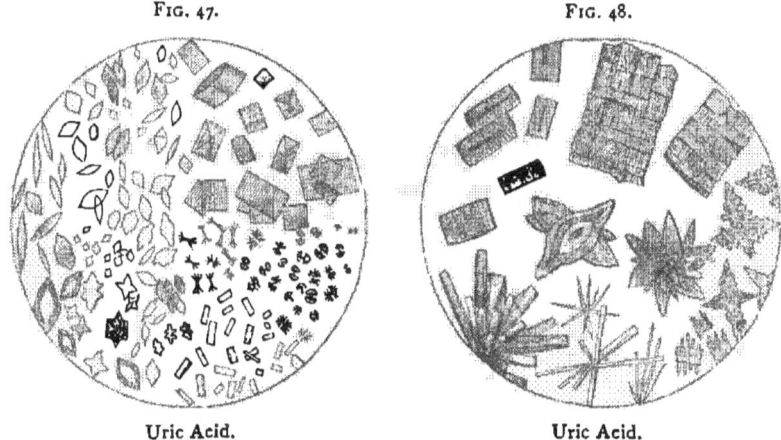

FIG. 47.   FIG. 48.

Uric Acid.   Uric Acid.

COLORING MATTERS.—Our unsatisfactory knowledge of these substances and their clinical significance is to be regretted, since some of them possess an importance next to albumin and sugar. The existence of at least two distinct substances have been demonstrated:—

1. *Urobilin* (*urohæmatin*), a brown resinous substance, derived from the coloring matter of the bile, and hence indirectly from the coloring matter of the blood.

It occurs in normal urine, and in larger quantity in the urine of patients suffering from any disease which causes disintegration of the blood corpuscles.

2. *Uro-indican* (*uroxanthin*) a substance closely related to, if not identical with, the glucoside *indican*, and, like that substance, it is capable of conversion into indigo-blue.

It seems to be a result of the fermentation of albuminous matters in the alimentary canal. It is therefore increased in obstructive troubles of the bowels, and in certain diseases characterized by impairment of general nutrition.

To estimate the coloring matters, put some urine in a beaker and render it strongly acid with nitric or hydrochloric acid. Let it stand six hours for the pigments to be liberated. Then note the depth of color by transmitted light.

PHOSPHATES.—The phosphates are derived mainly from the food, but to some extent also from oxidation of phosphorized tissues:—

1. *Earthy Phosphates* (Ca and Mg).—Being soluble only in acid

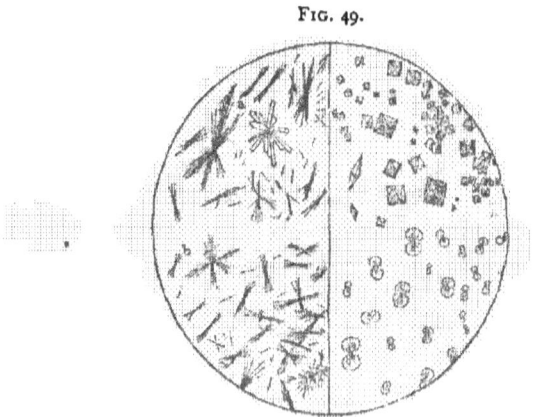

FIG. 49.

Urates.   Oxalate of Calcium.

solutions, the earthy phosphates are precipitated when the urine is made or becomes alkaline. Furthermore, being less soluble in warm than cold urine, heat often precipitates them, as in the heat test for albumin. Deposits of calcium and magnesium phosphates are generally amorphous, and may be distinguished from the amorphous urates, (*a*) by absence of color and not gathering in mossy forms; (*b*) **by a drop of acetic acid added to the sediment on a glass slide under the microscope—phosphates dissolve, while urates gradually lose their base and assume the characteristic forms of uric acid.** In ammoniacal urine (alkaline fermentation) the ammonio-magnesian phosphate ($MgNH_4PO_4$), the so-called *triple phosphate*, is formed and deposited in large prismatic, coffin-lid crystals; sometimes, also, in ragged stellate or aborescent crystals, resembling those of snow. (Fig. 50.) In cases of cystitis this may occur within the bladder; hence other calculi often have one or more white layers of the mixed phosphates.

2. *Alkaline Phosphates.*—These constitute the greater portion of the phosphates, and are made up mainly of *acid sodium phosphate*, with traces of potassium phosphate. Being very soluble, they never form a precipitate.

Magnesian Test.—The phosphates are best detected and estimated by precipitation with a solution composed of magnesium sulphate, ammonium chloride, and aq. ammoniæ, each one part, and water eight parts. If the precipitate be thick and creamy, the phosphates

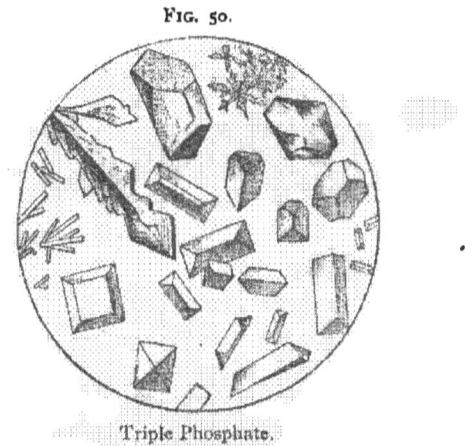

Fig. 50.

Triple Phosphate.

are abnormally increased; if it be milky, they are normal, and if translucent, diminished.

CHLORIDES.—These consist almost entirely of sodium chloride, the quantity depending mainly on what is taken in with the food. However, the chlorides are diminished or even disappear from the urine in many fevers, especially in pneumonia, much being eliminated by the sputa. Their reappearance in the urine is often the earliest indication of convalescence. Hence their detection and estimation are important.

Silver-Nitrate Test.—First add a few drops of nitric acid to prevent the precipitation of the phosphates. Then, on adding silver nitrate solution, only the chlorides will fall as a white precipitate of chloride of silver. If the precipitate be in curdy masses the chlorides are not diminished; if only a milkiness be produced, they are greatly diminished; and, if no cloudiness, they are entirely absent.

SULPHATES.—These consist mainly of sodium sulphate, with a little of the potassium salt. They are derived principally from the food, and in small amount from oxidation of albuminoid sulphurized tissues, especially in fevers. They are detected and estimated by precipitation with *barium chloride* or *nitrate*, first adding a little nitric or hydrochloric acid to hold the phosphates in solution. If the precipitate be creamy the sulphates are increased; if milky, normal, and if translucent, diminished.

ALBUMIN.—Under this head are included various proteid substances which, not being osmotic, appear in urine only in pathological conditions and functional disturbances. Many of the specific fevers, as pneumonia, typhoid, and diphtheria, produce albuminuria. Albuminous urine is apt to be of diminished transparency from presence of tube casts, fat granules, epithelial cells, etc., and filtering is often necessary before applying the tests.

Heat Test.—A test-tube is one-third filled with the suspected urine and held in the flame of a spirit lamp, or over the chimney of an ordinary lamp, until it boils. If an opacity occurs it must be either *albumin* or *earthy phosphates*. If earthy phosphates, it clears up on addition of nitric acid, but if albumin, it is slightly increased.

Nitric-Acid Test.—This consists in underlaying the urine with nitric acid. Take a test-tube one-fourth full, and, holding it aslant, gently pour in an equal volume of the acid, allowing it to trickle down the inside of the tube and pass beneath the urine. Or the acid may be put in first and the urine added afterward. An opacity at the junction of the two liquids is either *albumin* or the *urates*. If urates, it clears up on heating, but if albumin, it is permanent.

Either the heat or nitric-acid test, singly, is unsatisfactory, but both performed together are conclusive. However, the following sources of error should be borne in mind: (*a*) If the urine be very alkaline and the amount of albumin small, heat will cause no opacity; (*b*) if only a drop or two of nitric acid be added, it may hold a small quantity of albumin in solution; (*c*) urea may be precipitated from a concentrated urine by nitric acid, but heat dissolves it; (*d*) decomposed urates containing ammonium carbonate effervesce on addition of an acid; (*e*) often after taking turpentine, copaiba, etc., nitric acid precipitates resin in yellowish flakes, redissolved on addition of alcohol.

Other Tests.—Many other substances, as alcohol and certain acids and mineral salts, coagulate albumin and are used as tests for that substance. But they are less used, less convenient, and no more accurate and conclusive than the two already given. Among them may be mentioned (*a*) picric acid, (*b*) potassio-mercuric iodide (KI 50 grs.—$HgCl_2$ 21 grs.), (*c*) sodium tungstate, (*d*) potassium ferrocyanide. These added in saturated solution form white clouds with albumin, provided the urine is first acidulated with citric acid. Strips of filter paper steeped in these chemicals and dried, or pellets, are sometimes carried for use at the bedside.

FIG. 51.

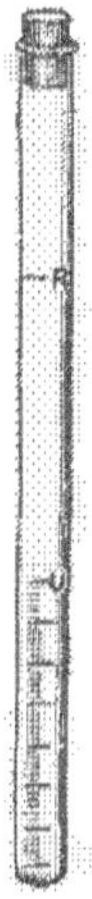

Quantitative Estimation.—During the progress of a disease it is often important to estimate the quantity of albumin. The exact method by drying and weighing the precipitated albumin is too laborious for the busy practitioner.

The easiest approximative method is to precipitate the albumin by heat, set it aside for twelve hours or until next visit, and then note the proportion of volume occupied by the precipitate—one-fourth, one-eighth, a trace, etc.

Esbach's Albuminometer (Fig. 51) is a graduated test-tube. Fill it to U with the urine and to R with the reagent, which is composed of 10 grammes of picric acid, 20 grammes of citric acid, and water sufficient to make a liter. Gently mix the liquids and set aside for twenty-four hours, to allow the precipitate to subside, the depth of which by the scale indicates the number of parts per thousand or grammes of albumin in a liter.

SUGAR (*Glucose*).—It has been proven (Dr. Pavy, 1879) that healthy urine contains traces of glucose, but quantities of clinical significance, and appreciable by the ordinary tests, are present only in glycosuria or diabetes, a pathological condition associated with some disturbance of the glycogenic function of the liver.

A temporary glycosuria may occur after the administration of anæsthetics and in certain brain lesions, especially those involving the floor of the fourth ventricle.

High specific gravity in a urine pale and copious, suggests sugar. Before testing, albumin, if present, should be removed by boiling and filtration.

Fermentation Test.—Two vials—one for comparison, the other for

PART III.—THE URINE.

fermentation—are partly filled with the urine. Into one is put a bit of baker's yeast about the size of a pea. Both vials are loosely plugged with some pervious material, as cotton, and set aside where they will keep warm (60° or 70° F.) until next day or next visit. If sugar be present, fermentation will occur in the vial treated with yeast, and CO_2 bubbles up and passes off through the cotton plug, and on taking the specific gravity of each, there will be a difference due to the loss of sugar in the vial fermented.

Alkali Test.—Boil the urine with liquor potassæ or sodæ, and if glucose be present it will be oxidized and form a molasses-like coloration, the depth of which indicates the amount of sugar present. On adding nitric acid a molasses-like odor is developed and the coloration discharged.

Alkali-Copper Test.—This depends on the power glucose has of reducing the cupric to the cuprous oxide. There are several methods of performing this test:—

(1) *Trommer's.* A drop or two of a weak (about 1 to 30) solution of cupric sulphate is added to an inch of urine in a test-tube, and then an equal bulk of liquor potassæ or sodæ. Immediately there falls, in addition to the earthy phosphates, a bluish precipitate. If sugar is present, this precipitate dissolves on agitation, forming a blue solution, which, on boiling, deposits a yellow, orange, or red precipitate of cuprous oxide. (See p. 86.)

(2) *Fehling's.* This differs from Trommer's in the addition of tartaric acid or some tartrate to dissolve the blue precipitate. Furthermore, the ingredients are in definite proportion, so as to make the solution available for quantitative analysis. Below are given the two formulæ in general use, one in the French and the other in the English measures:—

	Fehling's Solution.	Pavy's Solution.
Cupric Sulphate,	34.64 grams.	320 grains.
Potassium Tartrate,	173.20 grams.	640 grains.
Caustic Potash,	80.00 grams.	1280 grains.
Water,	1 liter.	20 ounces.

On standing a long time this solution is apt to spoil, the tartaric acid being converted into racemic acid, which, like glucose, will deoxidize the cupric oxide. Hence, it is best to make the solution in two separate parts, the cupric sulphate with one-half the water and the tartrate and caustic potash with the other half. For use, mix equal parts, forming

Fehling's solution fresh. A convenient amount should be put in a test-tube and boiled alone for a few seconds. If it remains clear it is good, and the urine may then be added gradually. Either immediately, or when the heat is reapplied, if sugar be present, the reddish precipitate will appear. Heat should not be applied longer than a minute, for prolonged boiling can cause the reduction of the copper oxide by various other organic substances found in the urine.

(3) *Haines'* differs from Fehling's in that glycerine is used instead of the tartrate, and the solution does not spoil.

Alkali-Bismuth Test.—(1) To some urine in a test-tube add a pinch of bismuth subnitrate and then an equal volume of liquor potassæ. Boil about two minutes. If sugar be present, the bismuth will be reduced and deposited as a black metallic mirror on the sides and bottom of the tube. (2) A bismuth test solution corresponding to Fehling's is made by warming a scruple each of bismuth subnitrate and tartaric acid in two ounces of water, and adding liquor potassæ until a clear solution is obtained. This boiled with a urine containing glucose gives the black bismuth precipitate.

The elements of the foregoing tests put up in pellets and tablets, while more convenient, are less reliable and spoil sooner than the solution.

Picric-Acid Test.—This is an extremely delicate test for glucose, and has the practical advantage of being as good a test for albumin. To the suspected urine add an equal volume of a saturated solution of picric acid. A cloudy precipitate indicates albumin. Next add a few drops of liquor potassæ and warm gently. A *deep red* color indicates sugar, though a lighter coloration may occur in urine free from glucose.

Indigo-Carmine Test.—To the urine add a solution of indigo-carmine rendered alkaline by sodium carbonate. Boil, and if sugar be present the blue mixture changes to violet-red and yellow. On agitation oxygen is absorbed from the air, and the above changes of color are reversed.

Quantitative.—(1) *Fermentation.* Each degree of specific gravity lost in fermenting represents one grain of sugar to the ounce of the twenty-four hours' urine.

(2) *Fehling's. Two hundred minims of the solution is decolorized by one grain of sugar.* Two hundred minims (grains) of the test solution are measured off into a small flask, diluted with twice its bulk

of water, and gently boiled (Fig. 52). A graduated burette (also shown in figure) is then filled to zero with the urine. To the boiling test solution the urine is added drop by drop till the blue color is discharged. By the graduations on the burette the quantity of urine added is easily read. As that represents one grain of sugar, the amount of sugar in the entire urine is easily calculated.

(3) *Alkali Test.* A light yellow indicates one per cent.; dark amber, two per cent.; sherry wine, three per cent.; dark Jamaica rum, five per cent., and dark, almost opaque, ten per cent.

BLOOD gives to urine a smoky hue, or even a dark-brown color.

FIG. 52.

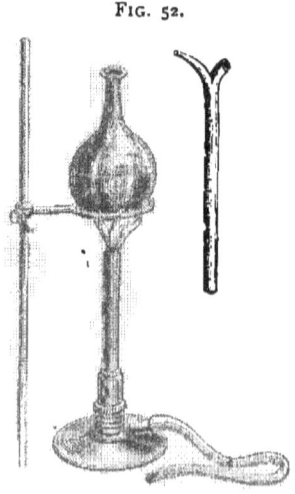

Hæmaturia (blood in urine) may occur as the result of (*a*) some disease or injury in the genito-urinary tract, as acute nephritis, calculus, parasites, cancer, wounds, etc.; (*b*) a depraved condition of the blood, as in scurvy, purpura, and eruptive fevers; (*c*) a disturbance of the renal circulation, as in mental emotions, malarial paroxysms, and cardiac obstructions.

If the urine be acid, the blood corpuscles retain their shape for several days and are easily recognized by the microscope. They appear as amber-colored, biconcave disks, either single or laid in rows, like piles of coin. Owing to the biconcavity of the corpuscles, their centres and peripheries alternate in brightness and shadow, as the object-glass is made to approach or recede. Their color and smaller size also serve to distinguish them from pus corpuscles. In doubtful cases a minute drop of blood, taken from the finger with a needle, may be used for comparison. After urine containing blood has stood for some time, the corpuscles lose their regular outline and become shriveled and angular. (See *a* in figure.) If the corpuscles be disintegrated and dissolved, we must *test* for *blood-coloring matters*.

The spectroscope offers the best means for their detection, but as physicians are seldom provided with that instrument, the following is the *test:* Place the urine in a test-tube and shake up with equal volumes of tincture of guaiacum and ozonized ether or old oil of tur-

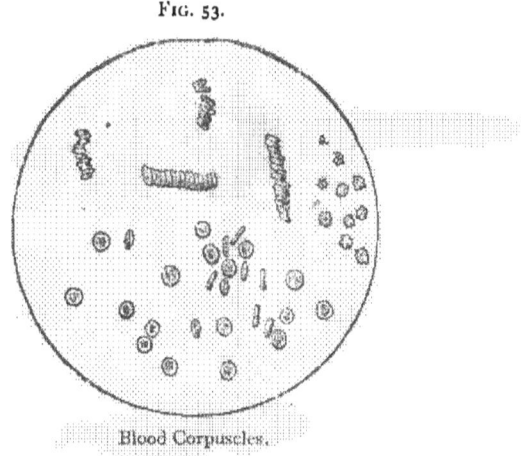

FIG. 53.

Blood Corpuscles.

pentine. If blood-coloring matters are present, the precipitated resin is *blue*, instead of a dirty greenish yellow.

BILE.—Urine containing bile is yellow, froths on shaking, and a rag dipped in it and dried is permanently yellow.

1. *Test for Bile-coloring Matters.**—(*a*) Underlay the urine with yellow nitric acid or a mixture of nitric and sulphuric acids; or the urine and acid may be placed adjacent on a white plate. In either

---

* Bilirubin oxidizes so easily that icteric urine often gives only the green coloration, or, if kept long, fails to respond at all. Hence, if fresh icteric urine cannot be obtained and bile urine must be prepared for demonstration, fresh bile from a recently killed animal, and not the inspissated, must be used.

method there occurs, at the junction of the liquids, a play of colors, *green* being prominent and characteristic; (*b*) overlay the urine with tincture of iodine. At junction of the liquids a green color will appear.

2. *Test for Bile Acids.*—Add a few grains of cane sugar or glucose to the urine and underlay it with sulphuric acid. At the junction of the liquid a *reddish-purple* color appears. As other substances than the bile acids may produce this reaction, we must, in cases of doubt, evaporate the urine to dryness, extract with alcohol, precipitate with ether, and redissolve in distilled water, and then apply the test as above.

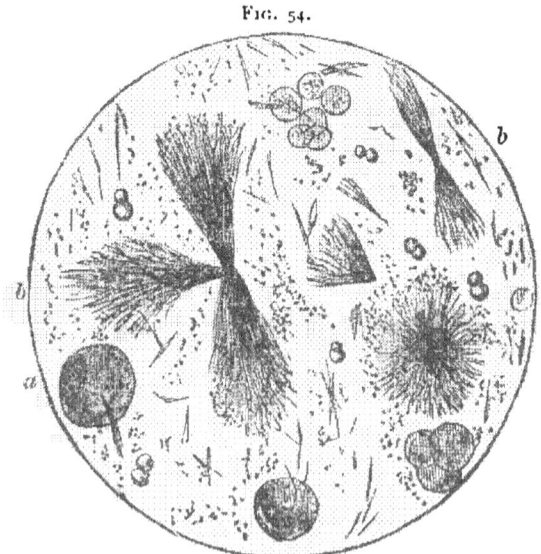

Fig. 54.

Leucin Spherules and Tyrosin Needles.

LEUCIN AND TYROSIN occur only in bile urine, for they attend destructive liver disease, especially acute, yellow atrophy and phosphorus-poisoning. They form yellowish crystalline deposits (Fig. 54) —leucin as spherules, with concentric striæ, and tyrosin as sheaf-like bundles of fine needles.

CYSTIN is a rare urinary sediment, a yellowish deposit of hexagonal plates (Fig. 55), not dissolved by heat or acetic acid but readily by ammonia. It is a highly sulphurized body whose formation in the system is obscure. It sometimes forms calculi.

CARBONATE OF CALCIUM is a very rare deposit in human, but abundant in the urine of cattle. It occurs in small spherules (Fig. 56) sometimes coalescing; acetic acid dissolves it with effervescence.

HIPPURIC ACID (*Horse-uric Acid*) largely replaces uric acid in the urine of herbivorous animals, and to some extent in that of man, especially after a vegetable diet. It occurs in pointed, four-sided prisms and acicular crystals, insoluble in acetic acid but soluble in alcohol. (Fig. 56.)

CALCIUM OXALATE *occurs* in extremely small amounts in normal urine, but more abundantly in the so-called oxalic diathesis and in certain forms of dyspepsia, or after eating rhubarb or other things

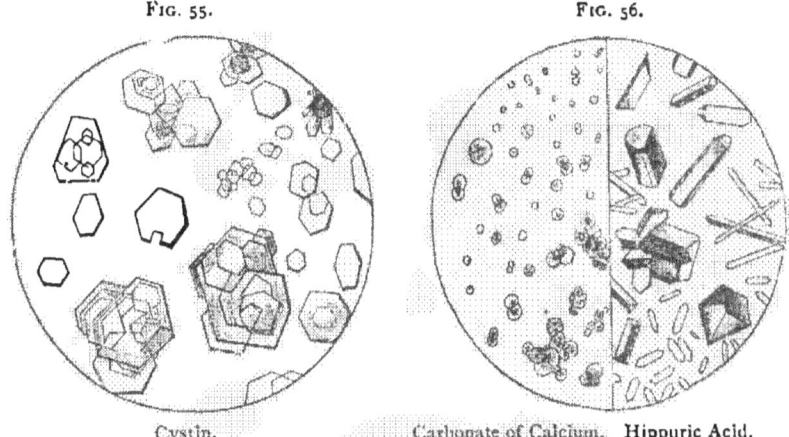

FIG. 55. FIG. 56.

Cystin.   Carbonate of Calcium. Hippuric Acid.

containing it. If persistently present it may form a (mulberry) calculus. It occurs in both acid and alkaline urine, and always as a light delicate precipitate, which under high powers is seen to consist of small, brilliant octahedral crystals, but sometimes dumb-bells. (Fig. 49.) In certain aspects the smaller octahedra appear as squares crossed by two bright diagonal lines.

FAT in such quantities as to float on the urine generally comes from the introduction of a catheter or from foreign admixture. Fatty degeneration of kidney, or leakage of a lymph vessel, or the opening of an abscess into the urinary tract may cause fat in the urine. It occurs as minute, highly refracting globules of various sizes (see *a* in Fig. 57), but sometimes, especially in chylous urine, in more intimate

PART III.—THE URINE.

emulsion (as at *b*), the globules appearing under the microscope as mere specks. Fat may be recognized by its dissolving on addition of ether.

MUCUS AND PUS.—Mucus is a normal constituent of urine. It is a transparent fluid, and would be invisible but for the mucus corpuscles, epithelium and other sediments entangled in it. Though closely related to albumin, mucin is coagulated by acetic acid and not by heat. Mucus is increased by irritation of the urinary tract, but as inflammation supervenes albumin appears and the urine is purulent. The mucus and pus corpuscles present the same appearance under the microscope as other leucocytes, viz.: rounded, colorless, very granu-

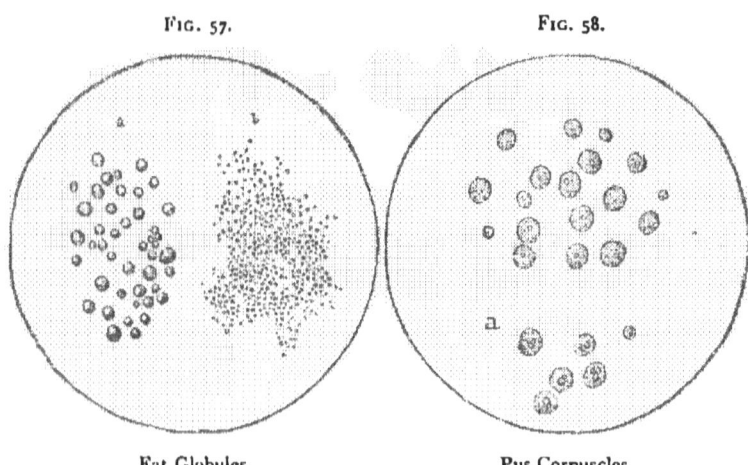

FIG. 57.   FIG. 58.

Fat Globules.   Pus Corpuscles.

lar cells, a little larger than red blood corpuscles. (Fig. 58.) If the urine be greatly diluted, or, better, treated with acetic acid, the cells swell up, lose their granular appearance, become transparent, and show their nuclei (*a* in Fig. 58). The pus cell oftener than the mucus corpuscle has more than one nucleus. Pus may be distinguished from mucus: (1) It is always attended with albumin; (2) (Donne's test) treated with an alkali it forms a gelatinous mass; (3) hydrogen peroxide causes marked effervescence with pus.

EPITHELIUM in the urine may come from any part of the genito-urinary tract. The accompanying cut shows the typical forms of cells coming from various situations. It is generally impossible to locate the origin of an epithelial cell beyond the vagina and bladder, for their distinctive differences, but slight at best, are rendered still fainter by maceration in the urine. *Renal* epithelium comes from the uriniferous tubules, and are rounded and granular, and, unlike pus cells, they show their nuclei without acetic acid. They are usually associated with albumin and tube casts (Fig. 60), and therefore point to kidney disease.

TUBE CASTS.—In hemorrhage from or inflammation of the kidney

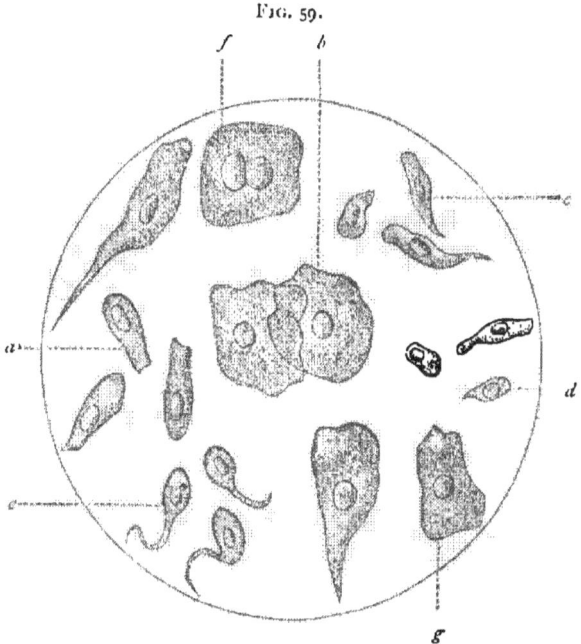

(*a*) Epithelium from the human urethra; (*b*) vagina; (*c*) prostate; (*d*) Cowper's glands; (*e*) Littre's glands; (*f*) female urethra; (*g*) bladder.

the urine usually contains microscopic casts or moulds of the uriniferous tubules formed by exudation into the tubule of coagulable material, which afterward contracts, becomes loose, and is washed out with the urine. As they imbed and bring away epithelial cells, granular matter, fat globules, blood disks, etc., they are a valuable index to the condition of the tubules. (1) *Epithelial* casts (see upper portion of figure) are those bearing renal epithelium. They indicate desquamative nephritis, (2) *Hyaline* casts (shown in left-hand part of figure) are transparent and comparatively free from entangled material. They come from tubules whose epithelium is sound and adherent or from those bereft of epithelium. In the latter case they are more solid in appearance (*waxy casts*) and indicate serious nephritis. (3) *Granular* casts are opaque from presence of granular *débris*. (4) *Fatty* casts (see larger cast in figure) are such as carry oil globules, either free or contained in epithelial cells. They are proof of fatty degeneration of the kidney. (5) *Blood* casts contain blood corpuscles, and show that the hæmaturia is of renal origin.

SPERMATOZOA occur in urine as a result of spermatorrhœa, noctur-

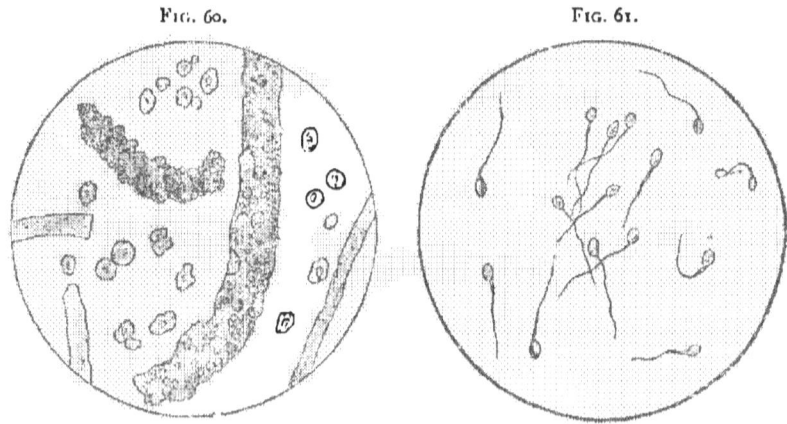

FIG. 60.   FIG. 61.

Epithelial Cells and Tube Casts.   Spermatozoa.

nal emissions, or coitus. They are liable to escape observation, for they subside slowly, and are very small and transparent. Under a high power they are seen to consist of a small oval cell with a tail-like prolongation. Their tadpole-like appearance is shown in Fig. 61. They are motionless in urine, and remain for days unaltered.

MICROÖRGANISMS.—Urine being a solution of organic matters becomes as soon as voided a ready medium for the growth of the lower forms of life, the germs of which get in from the air or unclean vessels. Besides various others we may mention: (1) *Yeast fungus* (shown on page 113) is seen during its sporule stage as transparent oval cells, sometimes arranging themselves in branches. It grows only in saccharine urine, though spores closely resembling it are seen

144   ESSENTIALS OF CHEMISTRY.

in acid urine containing neither sugar nor albumin. (2) *Sarcina* is a fungus seldom found in urine, but more frequently in matters vomited during certain diseases of the stomach. The cells are arranged in cubes, resembling bales bound with cross-bands. The sarcinæ shown at *a* in figure are from the urine, those at *b* from vomited matters.

3. *Bacteria (little rods).* This is the general term given to the minute moving organisms invariably present in putrefying animal and vegetable matter. They consist of simple cells filled with a colorless fluid and presenting several varieties of form: (*a*) *Micrococci* appear-

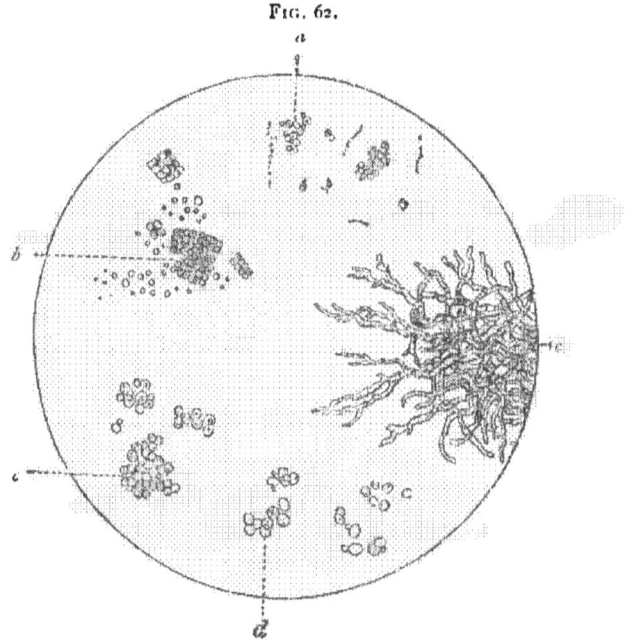

Fig. 62.

(*a*) Micrococci in short chains and groups; (*b*) sarcinæ; (*c*) fungi from acid fermentation, (*d*) yeast cells from diabetic urine; (*e*) mycelium of a fungus.

ing as trembling points, distinguished from other particles by their progressive motion; (*b*) *Rods* about the length of the diameter of blood disks, sometimes at rest, but usually vibrating across the field; (*c*) *Vibriones*, consisting of several rods joined together and moving with greater rapidity; and (*d*) *Zoögleæ*, aggregations of bacteria held together by gelatinous material and resembling masses of amorphous urates or phosphates. These various forms are shown in Fig. 41 and 42. Bacteria not only cause decomposition outside, but may set it up in urine while yet within the bladder, provided they be introduced from without. This may be done by dirty catheters and sounds, or they may work their way down the urethra in the pus of a gleet. The ammoniacal fermentation thus set up soon induces cystitis.

Extraneous bodies, such as hair, wool, or fragments of feathers, are often found in urinary deposits, and ludicrous mistakes have been made by observers not on their guard for such casual admixtures.

SEDIMENTS.—*The chemical examination* of unorganized urinary sediments is generally an easy matter, for they usually consist of urates, phosphates, calcium oxalate, or uric acid. Warm the sediment with the supernatant urine, it dissolves—*urates.* If not, warm with acetic acid, it dissolves—*phosphates.* If not, warm with hydrochloric acid, it dissolves—*calcium oxalate.* If not, it is *uric acid,* which may be confirmed by the murexid test.

URINARY CALCULI.—Urinary calculi (*calculus,* a pebble) are composed of urinary sediments which have gathered around some nucleus (usually calcium oxalate or uric-acid crystals, or some foreign body) within the bladder, and being slowly deposited, particle upon particle and layer upon layer, the concretion becomes as hard as stone. The concretion often consists of successive layers of different sediments deposited during varying conditions of the urine.

The qualitative analysis of calculi is easy. Saw the stone through the middle and see whether it be composed of the same material throughout or of successive layers of different sediments. If the former, take the sawdust; if the latter, chip off a specimen from a single layer. But this should be pulverized *very fine* (for it is dissolved much less readily than fresh sediments), and then test by means of heat, acetic and hydrochloric acids, just as other sediments.

The following method is easier in practice:—

I. Heat to redness on a piece of platinum foil. If no residue, see II; if a residue, see III.

II. To a fresh portion apply the murexid test. If it responds it is *ammonium urate* or *uric acid;* if it does not respond it is *cystin* or *xanthin,* see IV.

III. To the residue, when cool, add hydrochloric acid. If it effervesces it is an *oxalate* or *urate,* which may be determined by the murexid test; if it does not effervesce it is a *phosphate.*

IV. Dissolve some of the powder in nitric acid. If the solution is yellow it is *xanthin;* if dark brown it is *cystin.*

TABLE OF METRIC MEASURES.

MEASURES OF LENGTH.

1 Millimetre	=	0.001 of a metre.	
1 Centimetre	=	0.010 of a metre.	
1 Decimetre	=	0.100 of a metre	= about 4 inches.
1 **Metre**	=	**1.000 Metre**	= 39.37 inches.
1 Decametre	=	10.000 metres.	
1 Hectometre	=	100.000 metres.	
1 Kilometre	=	1000.000 metres	= about ⅝ of a mile.
1 Myriametre	=	10,000.000 metres	= about 6⅓ miles.

MEASURES OF SURFACE.

1 Centiare	=	1 Square metre	= about 1¼ square yards.
1 Are	=	100 Square metres.	
1 Hectare	=	10,000 Square metres	= about 2½ acres.

MEASURES OF VOLUME.

1 Cubic centimetre	=	0.001	of a litre.
1 Litre (cubic decimetre)	=	1000.	cubic centimetres.
1 Cubic metre	=	1000.	cubic decimetres.
1 Cubic metre	=	1000.	litres, or 1 kilolitre.
1 Cubic metre	=	1	stere.

MEASURES OF WEIGHT.

1 Milligramme	=	0.001 of a gramme	= about 1/64 of a grain.
1 Centigramme	=	0.010 of a gramme.	
1 Decigramme	=	0.100 of a gramme.	
1 **Gramme**	=	**1.000 Gramme**	= about 15½ grains.
1 Decagramme	=	10.000 grammes.	
1 Hectogramme	=	100.000 grammes.	
1 Kilo(gramme)	=	1000.000 grammes	= about 2¼ lbs.
1 Tonneau	=	1000. Kilos	= about 1 ton.

INDEX.

Absolute weight, 10
Acetanilide, 117
Acetic acid, 109
Acetic aldehyde, **108**
Acid acetic, 109
   antimonic, 54
   antimonious, 54
   arsenic, 49, 50
   arsenious, 49, 50
   benzoic, 109
   boric or boracic, 76
   chloric, **33**
   chlorous, **33**
   chromic, **79**
   citric, **110**
   cyanic, 61
   formic, 110
   gallic, 110
   hippuric, 140
   hydriodic, 31
   hydrobromic, 31
   hydrochloric, 31, 32
   hydrocyanic, 60
   hydroferricyanic, 61
   hydrofluoric, 31
   hydrosulphuric, 35
   hypochlorous, 33
   hyponitrous, 44
   lactic, 110
   lithic (see **Uric**), **129**
   malic, 110
   meconic, 119
   muriatic, 31
   myronic, 115
   nitric, 45
   nitrohydrochloric, 10
   nitromuriatic, 30
   nitrous, **45**
   oleic, 107
   orthophosphoric, **48**
   osmic, 93
   oxalic, 110
   palmitic, 107
   perchloric, 33
   phosphoric, 49
   picric, 110
   plumbic, 56
   prussic, 60
   pyrogallic, 111
   pyrophosphoric, **48**
   salicic, 56
   salicylic, 111

Acid, sodium phosphate, **123**, **132**
   stannic, 56
   stearic, 107
   succinic, 111
   sulphocarbolic, 104
   sulphocyanic, 61
   sulphuric, 39
   sulphurous, 37
   tannic, 111, 115
   tartaric, 111
   uric, 129
   valerianic, **111**
Acid salts, 69
Acids, definition **of, 16, 22**
   fatty, **107**
   organic, 109
Acidulous radical, **27**
Aconitine, 119
Analytical table, 94, 95
Affinity, chemical, 25
Aging of liquors, 103
Air, 41
Albumin, 116, 133
Alcohol, 101, 102
   amylic, 103
   ethylic, **102**
   glycerylic, **104**
   mannityl, **105**
   methylic, **101**
   phenylic, 104
   radicals, 101
   vinic, 102
   wood, 101
Aldehydes, 101, **108**
Ale, 103
Algaroth, powder of, 54
Alkalies, metals of the, 65
Alkaline earth metals, 71
Alkaline group, 65
Alkaloids, 118
Alloys, 62
Allotropic **forms,** 56
Allylsulphocyanate, **115**
Aluminium, 76
   bronze, 76
   chloride, 76
   silicates, 77
   sulphate, 76
Alum, 76
Amalgam, 62
Amides, 117
Amines, 117

INDEX.

Ammonia, 42
Ammoniac, 100
Ammoniated mercury, 89
Ammonio-chloride of mercury, 89
Ammonio citrate of iron, 84
  ferric alum, 77
  magnesium phosphate, 72
  nitrate of silver, 52
  sulphate of copper, 52
  tartrate of iron, 84
Ammonium, 66
  alum, 77
  amalgam, 66
  carbonate, 67
  hydrate, 66
  hydrosulphide, 67
  nitrate, 44
  nitrite, 41
Amygdalin, 61, 115
Amyl acetate, 104
  hydrate, 103
  nitrite, 106
Amylic alcohol, 103
Amyloses, 112
Amylum, 112
Analysis, 21
  acidulous radicals, 94
  definition of, 21
  metallic radicals, 94
Aniline, 117
Animal charcoal, 56
Antidote, definition of, 51
Antidotes to acids, 73
  to alkalies, 67
  to alkaloids, 118
  to antimony, 55
  to arsenic, 51
  to barium, 75
  to carbolic acid, 104
  to copper, 87
  to cyanides, 61
  to lead, 65
  to mercury, 90
  to oxalic acid, 110
  to silver, 92
  to sulphuric acid, 40
Antifebrin, 117
Antimonious chloride, 54
  hydride, 54
  oxychloride, 54
  oxide, 54
  sulphide, 54
Antimoniuretted hydrogen, 54
Antimony, 53
Antimony and potassium tartrate, 54
Antimony, butter of, 54
Antimonyl, 54
Antipyrine, 118
Antiseptics, 42
Antizymotics, 42
Apomorphine, 119
Apparent weight, 10
Aqua, 20
  ammonia, 66
  ammoniæ fortior, 66
  chlori, 29
  destillata, 23
  fortis, 45

Arbutin, 116
Argenti nitras, 91
Argol, 111
Arsenic, 49, 50
  acid, 49, 50
  oxide, 50
  pentoxide, 50
  toxicology of, 50
  white, 50
Arsenious acid, 49, 50
  hydride, 49
  iodide, 49
  sulphide, 49
Arseniuretted hydrogen, 49
Arsine, 49
Artificial parchment, 112
Asafœtida, 100
Asbestos, 62
Atmosphere, 41
Atomic theory, 12
  weight, 13
Atoms, 13
Atropine, 119
Auric chloride, 92

Babbitt's metal, 54
Bacteria, 120-144
Baking powders, 70
Balsam of Peru, 100
Balsams, 100
Barium, 75
  chromate, 75
Bases, 22
Basylous radicals, 27
Beer, 103
Beet sugar, 113
Bengal light, 75
Benzine, 98
Benzoic acid, 100
Benzoine, 100
Bichromates, 79
Bile in urine, 138
Bilirubin, 138
Bismuth, 55
  ammonio-citrate, 55
  nitrate, 55
  oxynitrate, 55
  subcarbonate, 55
  subnitrate, 55
Bismuthyl, 54
Black lead, 56
  oxide of manganese, 80
Bleaching, 24, 38, 74
  powder, 74
Blood casts, 143
  in urine, 137
Blue ointment, 87
  pill, 87
  vitriol, 85
Bluestone, 85
Boroglyceride, 76
Borax, 76
Boric acid, 76
Boron, 76
Brandy, 103
Brass, 77
Brimstone, 35

INDEX. 149

Britannia, 54
British gum, 113
Bromides, test for, 30
Bromine, 28
Bromum, 28
Bronze aluminium, 76
Brucine, 119
Butter of antimony, 54
Butyl, 101

Cadavarine, 120
Cadmium, 79
Cæsium, 63, 71
Caffeine, 119
Calcium, 73
    carbonate, 73, 140
    chloride, 73
    hydrate, 73
    oxalate, 74, 140
    oxide, 73
    phosphate, 74
    sulphate, 74
Calculi, urinary, 145
Calomel, 88–89
Calx, 73
    chlorata, 74
Camphor, monobromated, 100
Camphors, 100
Cane sugar, 113
Caoutchouc, 100
Caramel, 103
Carat fine, 92
Carbamide, 117
Carbazotic acid, 110
Carbolic acid, 104
Carbohydrates, 112
Carbon, 56
    dioxide, 57
    disulphide, 57
    group, 56
    monoxide, 57
Carbonic acid, 56, 57
Carburetted hydrogen, 99
Casein, 116
Catalysis, 18, 26, 105
Caustic ammonia, 66
    potash, 70
Cellulin, 112
Celluloid, 112
Cellulose, 112
Centimeter, cubic, 147
Cerium, 77
Chalk, 73
Charcoal, 56
    animal, 56
Chemical action, 9
    affinity, 25
Chemistry, definition of, 9
    inorganic, 15
    organic, 97
Chinoline, 118
Chloral, 108
    hydrate, 109
Chloralum, 76
Chloride of gold, 92
    of lime, 74
Chlorides in urine, 132

Chlorides, tests for, 132
Chlorinated lime, 74
Chlorine, 28
    group, 28
    oxides, 32
Chloroform, 106
Choke damp, 57
Cholesterine, 108
Choline, 120
Chondrin, 116
Chromates, 79
Chrome yellow, 64
Chromic acid, 79
Chromium, 79
    trioxide, 79
Cider, 103
Cinchona alkaloids, 119
Cinchonicine, 119
Cinchonidine, 119
Cinchonine, 119
Cinnabar, 90
Citric acid, 110
Citrine ointment, 88
Classification of elements, 15
Clay, 62
Coal, 56
    mineral, 56
Cobalt, 85
Cocaine, 119
Codeine, 119
Coin, 91, 92
Colchicine, 119
Collodion, 112
Colocynthin, 116
Coloring matters, urinary, 130
Combining weight, 13
Combustible, 18
Combustion, 18
    supporter of, 18
Compounds, 11
Concentrated lye, 69
Coniine, 119
Copal, 100
Copper, 85
    ammonia-sulphate, 52
    arsenite, 52
    black oxide, 86
    group, 85
    suboxide, 86
Copperas, 82
Corals, 73
Corrosive sublimate, 89
Cotton, 112
Crab orchard salts, 72
Cream of tartar, 69
Creasote, 105
Creatine, 120
Creatinine, 120
Creta preparata, 73
Crystallization, water of, 21
Cupric hydrate, 86
    oxide, 86
    subacetate, 86
    sulphate, 85
Cuprous oxide, 86
Cyanates, 61
Cyanic acid, 61
Cyanide, mercuric, 60

INDEX.

Cyanides, compound, 61
Cyanogen, 60
Cystin, 139

Davy's method for urea, 127
Decantation, 73
Decay, 114
Deliquesce, 21
Deodorizers, 42
Deposits, urinary, 145
Dew point, 42
Dextrin, 113
Diabetic sugar, 114
  urine, 134
Dialysis, 83
Dialyzed iron, 83
Dialyzer, 83
Diamond, 56
Diastase, 114
Didymium, 75
Diffusion, 60
  gases, 60
  liquids, 60
Digitalin, 116
Disinfectants, 42
Distillation, 23
Donne's test for pus, 141
Donovan's solution, 49
Doremus' method for urea, 128
Drummond light, 17
Dynamite, 104

Earths, metals of the, 75
Earthy phosphates, 122, 131, 133
Effloresces, 21
Elaterin, 116
Electrolysis, 25
Electro-positive and negative, 24
Elements, 11
  classification of, 15
  groups of, 15
Emplastrum plumbi, 63
Emulsin, 115
Epithelial casts, 142
Epithelium, 141
Epsom salts, 72
Equation, 14
Erbium, 75
Esbach's albuminometer, 134
Essential oils, 99
Etching, 32
Ether, 105
  chloric, 106
  hydrobromic, 106
  hydrochloric, 106
  nitrous, 106
  ozonized, 24
  sulphuric, 105
Ethers, compound, 101, 105
  simple, 101, 105
Ethyl bromide, 106
  aldehyde, 108
  chloride, 106
  hydrate, 102
  nitrite, 106
  oxide, 105

Ethylic alcohol, 102
Evaporation, 11
Extraneous bodies in urine, 145

Fat in urine, 140
Fatty casts, 143
Fats, 107
Fehling's test, 135
  solution, 136
Fermentation, acid, 123
  alkaline, 124
Ferments, 114
Ferri citras, 84
  carbonas saccharatus, 84
  et ammonii citras, 84
  et ammonii tartras, 84
  et potassii tartras, 84
  et quininæ citras, 84
  et strychniæ citras, 84
  pyrophosphas, 84
Ferric chloride, 81
  hydrate, 83
  nitrate, 84
  sulphate, 82
Ferricyanides, 61
Ferricyanogen, 61
Ferrocyanogen, 61
Ferrous chloride, 82
  carbonate, 84
  hydrate, 83
  iodide, 84
  sulphate, 82
  sulphide, 84
Ferrum redactum, 81
Fibrin, 116
Filtration, 73
Fixed oils, 107
Flint, 62
Flowers of sulphur, 35
Fluorides, tests for, 32
Fluorine, 28
Fluorspar, 28
Fluxes, 81
Flystone, 85
Formic acid, 110
Formulæ, 14
Fowler's method for urea, 128
  solution, 50
Fruit essences, artificial, 104
Fungi, 122
Fusel oil, 103

Galena, 63
Gallic acid, 110
Galls, oak, 111
Galvanized iron, 77
Gas, definition of, 10
  illuminating, 57
  laughing, 44
  marsh, 99
Gasoline, 98
Gelatine, 116
Gentianin, 116
German silver, 85
Germicides, 42
Glass, 62

Globulin, 116
Glucose, 114, 134
Glucosides, 115
Glycerine, 104
Glycerites, 104
Glycyrrhizin, 116
Glycerylic alcohol, 104
Glycogen, 113
Gold, 92
   leaf, 92
Goulard's extract, 63
Gramme, 147
Granular casts, 143
Grape sugar, 114
Graphite, 56
Gravity, specific, 10
Gray powder, 87
Green fire, 75
Green vitriol, 82
Group, alkaline, 65
   alkaline earths, 71
   carbon, 56
   chlorine, 28
   copper, 85
   hydrogen and oxygen, 15
   iron, 79
   nitrogen, 40
   zinc, 77
Guaiacol, 105
Guaiacum, tincture, 138
Gum resins, 100
Gums, 112
Gun cotton, 112
Gutta percha, 100
Gypsum, 74

Haines' test, 136
Hair dye, 111
Hartshorn, 43
   spirits of, 43
Homatropine, 119
Homologous series, 98
Hyaline casts, 143
Hydracids, 31
Hydrates, 22
Hydrargyri—
   chloridum mite, 88
   cum creta, 87
   iodidum rubrum, 88
      viride, 88
   oxidum flavum, 89
      rubrum, 89
   subsulphas flavus, 88
Hydrargyrum, 87
   cum creta, 87
Hydrobromic ether, 106
Hydrocarbons, 98
Hydrochloric ether, 106
Hydrocyanic acid, 60
Hydro-ferricyanic acid, 61
Hydro-ferrocyanic acid, 61
Hydrogen, 16
   carburetted, 99
   cyanide, 60
   dioxide, 24
   oxide, 20
   peroxide, 20

Hydrogen sulphide, 35
Hyoscyamine, 119
Hydrometer, 10
"Hypo," 33
Hyponitrous acid, 44
Hyposulphite of sodium, 38
Hyposulphites, 38
   "ic," 27
   "ide," 33

Ice, 20
Ignis fatuus, 47
Indestructibility, 9
India rubber, 100
Indican, 116, 130
Ink, black, 111
   indelible, 92
   sympathetic, 85
Inorganic chemistry, 15
Insolubility, influence of, 26
Insoluble chlorides, 91
Introduction, 9
Iodide of nitrogen, 41
   of starch, 1
Iodides, tests for, 32
Iodine, 28
Iodoform, 107
Iridium, 93
Iron, 81
   by hydrogen, 81
   cast, 81
   group, 79
   pig, 81
   reduced, 81
   salts (see Ferrous and Ferric), 81
   scale compounds of, 84
   wrought, 81
Isologous series, 98
Isomeric bodies, 99
Isomerism, 98
   "ite," 33

Jalapin, 116
Javellé water, 71

Kalium, 65
Kaolin, 77
Kerosene, 98
Kreatine, 129
Kreatinine, 129

Labarraque's solution, 71
Lac sulphuris, 35
Lactic acid, 110
Lana philosophica, 78
Lanolin, 108
Lanthanum, 75
Laughing gas, 44
Lead, 63
   acetate, 63
   carbonate, 64
   chloride, 64
   chromate, 64
   dioxide, 63

Lead, iodide, 64
 nitrate, 63
 oxide, 63
 plaster, 63
 puce, 63
 red, 63
 subacetate, 63
 sugar of, 63
 sulphate, 64
 sulphide, 64
 water, 63
 white, 64
Ledoyen's disinfectant fluid, 63
Leucin, 139
Leucomaines, 120
Lignin, 112
Lime (see Calcium), 73
 chloride, 73
 kilns, 73
 quick, 73
 slaked, 73
 water, 73
Limestone, 73
 magnesian, 71
Linen, 112
Linseed oil, 108
Liquid, definition of, 10
Liquor, 20-66
 acidi arseniosi, 50
 arsenii et hydrargyri iodidi, 49
 calcis, 73
 saccharatus, 73
 definition of, 20, 66
 ferri chloridi, 82
  nitratis, 84
  subsulphatis, 83
  tersulphatis, 83
 hydrargyri nitratis, 88
 iodi compositus, 30
 magnesii citratis, 72
 plumbi subacetatis, 63
 potassæ, 70
 potassii arsenitis, 50
Liter, 146
Litharge, 63
Lithium, 65
 urate, 65
Litmus, 67, 125
Lixiviation, 69
Lubricating oil, 99
Lugol's solution, 30
Lunar caustic, 91
Lustre, metallic, 62
Lye, 69

Magnesia, 72
 milk of, 72
Magnesian fluid, 49
 limestone, 71
Magnesium, 71
 carbonate, 72
 citrate, 72
 hydrate, 72
 oxide, 72
 phosphatis, 72
 sulphate, 72
Malic acid, 110

Malt, 114
Maltin, 114
Manganates, 80
Manganese, 80
 black oxide of, 80
 dioxide, 80
Manganous sulphate, 80
 sulphide, 80
Manna, 105
Mannite, 105
Mannityl alcohol, 105
Marble, 73
Marsh gas, 99
Marsh's test, 52
Mastic, 100
Matter, 9
Measures, 146
Meerschaum, 71
Menthol, 100
Mercurial ointment, 87
Mercuric ammonium chloride, 89
 chloride, 89
 cyanide, 60
 iodide, 88
 nitrate, 88
 oxide, 89
 sulphate, 88
 sulphide, 90
Mercurous chloride, 88
 iodide, 88
 nitrate, 88
 oxide, 89
 sulphate, 88
 sulphide, 89
Mercury, 87
 acid nitrate, 88
 ammoniated, 89
 bichloride, 89
 biniodide, 88
 black oxide, 89
 green iodide, 88
 mild chloride, 88
 oleate, 89
 proto-iodide, 88
 red iodide, 88
 red oxide, 89
 yellow oxide, 89
Metallic lustre, 62
Metals, 15, 62
Metaphosphoric acid, 48
Methane, 99
Methyl hydrate, 101
Methylated spirit, 102
Methylic alcohol, 101
Metric measures, 146
Micrococci, 144
Micrococcus urea, 124
Microörganisms, 22, 114, 143
Milk of magnesia, 72
 of sulphur, 35
 sugar, 114
Millimeter, 146
Mineral coal, 56
Molecules, 13
Molybdenum, 93
Monobromated camphor, 100
Monsel's solution, 83
Morphine, 119

INDEX.   153

Mother of vinegar, 114
Mucilage of starch, 113
Mucus, 122, 141
Mulberry calculus, 140
Murexid test, 130
Muscarine, 120
Mustard, 115
Mycoderma aceti, 109, 114
Myronic acid, 115
Myrrh, 100

Naphtha, 98
Narceine, 119
Narcotine, 119
Nascent state, 26
Natrium, 65
Negative radicals, **27, 28**
Neuridine, 120
Nitre, sweet **spirits of, 106**
Nickel, 85
Nicotine, 119
Nitrates, tests for, 46
Nitric acid, 45
Nitric oxide, 45
Nitrification, 45
Nitrite of amyl, 106
Nitrites, 45
Nitro-cellulose, 112
Nitrogen, 40
    dioxide, 45
    group, 40
    hydride, 42
    iodide of, 41
    monoxide, 44
    oxides, 44
    pentoxide, **45**
    tetroxide, 45
    trioxide, 45
Nitrogenous bodies, 116
Nitro-glycerine, 104
Nitrous acid, 43
    ether, 106
    oxide, **44**
Non-metals, 15
Nux vomica **alkaloids, 119**

Oïdium albicans, 114
Oil, fusel, 103
    linseed, 108
    of vitriol, 39
Oils, essential, 99
    fixed, **107**
    volatile, **99**
Oleic, 107
Oleo-resins, 100
Oleum terebinthinæ, 99
Opium alkaloids, **119**
Organic acids, 109
Organic chemistry, **97**
Organized bodies, 97
Orpiment, 49
Orthophosphoric acid, 48
Osmic acid, 93
Osmium, 93
"Ous," 27
Oxacids, 32

Oxalate of lime, **74**
Oxalic acid, 110
Oxidation, 18
Oxide, definition of, **18**
Oxidizing agents, 19
Oxychloride of antimony, **54**
Oxygen, 17
Oxygenated water, 20
Oxyhydrogen flame, **17**
Ozone, 19
    test for, **20**
Ozonized ether, **24**

Painters' colic, **65**
Pancreatin, 114
Paper, 112
Paraffine, 98
Paraldehyde, 108
Parchment, artificial, **112**
Paris green, 52
Pavy's solution, **135**
Pearl ash, 69
    white, 55
Pepsin, 114
"Per," 33
Perspiration, 11
Peru, balsam of, **100**
Petrolatum, 98
Petroleum, 98
Pewter, 55, 63
Phenates, 104
Phenacetine, 118
Phenol, 104
Phenyl alcohol, 104
    bisulphate, 105
Phenylamine, 117
Phosphates in urine, **131**
Phosphine, 47
Phosphoretted hydrogen, **47**
Phosphoric acid, **49**
Phosphorus, **45**
    hydride, 47
    oxides, 48
    pentoxide, **48**
Picric acid, 110
    test for glucose, 136
Physostigmine, 119
Pilocarpine, 119
Pilula hydrargyri, 87
Plaster-of-Paris, 74
Plasters, 108
Platinic chloride, **71, 93**
Platinum, 92
Plumbago, 56
Plumbic acid, **56**
Plumbum, 63
Poisoning by **chloroform, 107**
Porcelain, 77
Porter, 103
Port wine, 103
Potassium, 68
    acid carbonate, **69**
    bromide, 70
    bicarbonate, 69
    bichromate, 70
    bitartrate, 69
    carbonate, 69

154 INDEX.

Potassium chlorate, 17
  chromate, 79
  ferricyanide, 61
  ferrocyanide, 61
  hydrate, 70
  hypochlorite, 70
  iodate, 70
  iodide, 70
  manganate, 80
  permanganate, 80
  red chromate, 79
  sodium tartrate, 70
  sulpho-cyanate, 61
Potato starch, 112
Powder of Algaroth, 54
Precedence of affinities, 25
Precipitated chalk, 73
Principles, proximate and ultimate, 100
Propylamine, 117
Propyl, 101
Proteids, 116
Proximate analysis, 100
  principles, 100
Prussiate of potash, red, 61
  yellow, 61
Prussic acid, 60
Ptomaïnes, 119
Ptyalin, 114
Ptyalism, 90
Purification of water, 23
Pus in urine, 141
Putrefaction, 114
Putrescine, 120
Pyroligneous, 101
Pyrogallic acid, 111
Pyrophosphoric acid, 48

Quantivalence, 26
Quevenne's iron, 81
Quicklime, 73
Quicksilver, 87
Quinicine, 119
Quinidine, 119
Quinine, 119
Quinoidine, 119

Radicals, definition of, 24
  basylous, 27
  negative, 24
  positive, 27
  the alcohol, 101
Rancidity of fats, 128
Ratsbane, 50
Realgar, 49
Red fire, 75
Red prussiate of potash, 61
Reduced iron, 81
Reinsch's test, 52
Resina, 99
Resins, 99
Resorcin, 105
Respiration, 19
Rex magnus, 76
Rhigoline, 99
Rochelle salt, 70

Rock crystal, 62
Roll sulphur, 00
Rosin (see Resin), 99
Rubidium, 65, 71

Saccharoses, 113
Salicylic acid, 111
Salicin, 115
Salivation, 90
Salt, common, 31
Salts, acid, 69
  "bi," 69
  crab orchard, 72
  Epsom, 72
  normal, 69
  of tartar, 69
Sal volatile, 67
Samarium, 75
Sand, 62
Santonin, 116
Saponification, 108
Saponin, 116
Sarcina, 144
Scale compounds of iron,
Scandium, 75
Scheele's green, 52
Secretion of urine, 121
Sediments, urinary, 145
Selenium, 34
Sewer gas, 35
Shellac, 100
Sherry wine, 103
Silicates, 62
Silicic acid, 56, 62
Silicic oxide, 62
Silicon, 61
Silver, 91
  action of light on, 92
  ammonio-nitrate, 52
  arsenite, 52
  bromide, 92
  chloride, 91
  cyanide, 91
  german, 85
  group, 91
  iodide, 92
  nitrate, 91
  oxide, 91
Slaked lime, 73
Soaps, 108
Soapstone, 62
Soda water, 58
Sodio-ammonium, 66
Sodio-potassium tartrate, 70
Sodium, 67
  amalgam, 66
  borate, 76
  chloride, 67
  hypochlorite, 71
  hyposulphite, 38
  salicylate, 111
  sulphocarbolate, 105
Solder, 63
Solid, definition of, 10
Solanin, 116
Soluble glass, 62
Solution, Donovan's, 49

INDEX.

Solution, Labarraque's, 71
   rationale of, 21
Spasmotoxine, 120
Specific gravity, 10
   flask, 10
   weight, 10
Spectroscope, 138
Spermatozoa, 143
Spirit, methylated, 102
   pyroligneous, 101
Spirits, 66
   of hartshorn, 43
   of wine, 102
Spiritus ætheris nitrosi, 106
   ammoniæ, 66
   ammoniæ aromaticus, 66
   frumenti, 103
   vini gallici, **103**
Stannic acid, 56
   salts, 63
Stannous salts, 63
Stannum, 56
Starch, 112
Steam, 20
Steel, 81
Stereotyping metal, 55
Stibine, **54**
Stibium, **53**
Strontium, 75
Strychnine, 119
Styptic collodion, 112
Sublimation, 23
Sublimed sulphur, 35
Succinic acid, 111
Sugar, beet, 113
   cane, 113
   diabetic, **114**
   grape, 114
   in urine, 134
   milk, 114
   of lead, 63
Sulphates, tests for, 133
Sulphites, 38
Sulpho-cyanates, 61
Sulphur, 35
   dioxide, 37
   lotum, 35
   precipitatum, 35
   sublimatum, 35
   peroxide, 38
Sulphuretted hydrogen, 35
Sulphuric acid, 39
   ether, 105
Supporter of combustion, 18
Symbols, 13
Sympathetic ink, **85**
Synaptase, 115
Synthesis, 21
Syrupus calcii lacto-phosphatis, 74
   scillæ comp., 54
   simplex, 114

Table, analytical, for metals, 94
   analytical, for negative radicals, 95
   of elements, 12
   of metric measure, 146
   of solubilities, 96

Table of valences, 27
Tannic acid, 111
Tannin, 111, 115
Tartar, cream of, **69**
   emetic, 54
Tartaric acid, **111**
Tellurium, 34
Temperature, influence of, 25
Terebene, 99
Terminations, 27
Tersulphate of iron, 82
Tests, acidity, 67
   acidulous radicals, 95
   alcohol, 102
   alkali metals, 71
   alkaline earth metals, **75**
   alkalinity, 67
   ammonia, 44
   ammonium salts, 67
   antimony, **55**
   arsenic, 51
   barium, **75**
   bile, 138
   bile acids, 139
   bismuth, 55
   blood, 137
   boron, 76
   bromide, 32
   bromine, 32
   brucine, **119**
   cadmium, 79
   calcium, 75
   carbonates, 59
   carbon dioxide, 59
   carbonic acid, 59
   chlorides, 32
   chlorine, 32
   chloroform, 107
   chromates, 80
   cobalt, 85
   coloring matters, urinary, **130**
   copper, 86
   cyanides, **61**
   fats, 140
   fluorides, 32
   fluorine, 32
   gallic acid, 110
   glucose in urine, **134**
   hard water, 22
   heat, for albumen, **133**
   hydrocyanic acid, **61**
   hydrogen sulphide, 36
   iodides, 32
   iodoform, 107
   iodine, 32
   iron, 84
   lead, 64
   lithium, 66
   magnesian, **75**
   manganese, **80**
   Marsh's, 52–55
   mercury, 90
   metallic radical, 94
   morphine, 119
   murexid, 130
   nickel, 85
   nitrates, 46
   nitric acid, 46

INDEX.

Tests, nitrogenous bodies, 116
  organic matter in water, 23
  oxalic acid, 111
  oxygen, 18, 45
  ozone, 19
  phosphates, 133
  phosphoric acid, 49
  phosphorus, 47
  potassium, 71
  pus, 141
  pyrogallic acid, 111
  quinine, 119
  Reinsch's, 52
  salicylic acid, 111
  silver, 92
  sodium, 68
  starch, 113
  strychnine, 119
  strontium, 75
  sugar, 134
  sulphates, 40, 133
  sulphuric acid, 39
  tannic acid, 111
  urates, 129
  urea, 127
  uric acid, 130
  urinary calculi, 145
  urinary sediments, 145
  water in alcohol, 85
  zinc, 78
Tetanine, 120
Tetanotoxine, 120
Theine, 119
Theory, atomic, 12
Thrush, 114
Tin, 62
Tinct. ferri chloridi, 85
  iodi, 30
Tinctures, 66
Tin foil, 62
Tolu, 100
Torula cerevisiae, 114
Toxicology of arsenic, 50
Trichloraldehyde, 108
Trichlormethane, 106
Trimethylamine, 117
Triple phosphate, 131
Trommer's test, 135
Trypsin, 114
Tube casts, 142
Turpene, 99
Turpentine, 99
Turpeth mineral, 88
Type metal, 63
Typhotoxine, 120
Tyrotoxine, 120
Tyrosin, 139

Ultimate analysis, 100
  principals, 100
Unguentum antimonii, 54
  hydrargyri, 87
  nitratis, 88
Urates, 122, 130, 133
Urea, 117, 119, 126
  estimation of, 127
  nitrate, 127

Urea, quantitative analysis, 127
  tests for, 127
Uric acid, 129
Urinary calculi, 145
  sediments, 145
Urine, 121
  acid fermentation, 123
  alkaline fermentation, 124
  chemical constituents, 126
  color, 123
  coloring matters, 130
  fluidity, 122
  normal, 122
  odor, 123
  opacity, 122
  physical properties, 122
  quantity, 122
  reaction, 123
  specific gravity, 125
  transparency, 122
Urinometer, 125
Urobilin, 130
Urohæmatin, 130
Uroindican, 130
Uroxanthin, 130

Valence, 26
Valerian, 111
Valerianic acid, 111
Vaseline, 99
Veratrine, 119
Ventilation, 59
Verdigris, 86
Vermilion, 90
Vibriones, 145
Vinegar, 109
Vinum antimonii, 54
  rubrum, 103
  xericum, 103
Vitellin, 116
Vitriol, blue, 85
  green, 82
  oil of, 39
  white, 78
Volatile oils, 99
Volatility, influence of, 25
Vulcanized rubber, 100

Water, 20
  alkaline, 24
  chalybeate, 24
  carbonated, 23
  distilled, 23
  drinkable, 22
  gas, 20
  hard, 22, 74
  impure, test for, 23
  mineral, 23
  natural, 22
  of crystallization, 21
  oxygenated, 20
  potable, 22
  purification of, 23
  saline, 24
  sulphur, 24
  thermal, 24

INDEX. 157

Water-glass, 62
Waxy casts, 143
Weight, 9
   absolute, 10
   apparent, 10
Weights, atomic, 13
   combining, 13
   specific, 10
White arsenic, 50
   lead, 64
   precipitate, 89
   vitriol, 78
Whisky, 103
"Will-o'-the-wisp," 47
Wines, 103
Wood alcohol, 101
   naphtha, 101
   spirit, 101
Woody fibre, 112

Xanthin, 120, 145

Yeast, 114
   fungus, 143
Yellow chrome, 64
   prussiate of potash, 61
Ytterbium, 75
Yttrium, 75

Zinc, 77
   carbonate, 78
   chloride, 78
   oxide, 78
   sulphate, 78
   sulphide, 78
   white, 78
Zoogleæ, 144

CATALOGUE No. 7.   **JULY, 1890.**

A CATALOGUE
OF
BOOKS FOR STUDENTS.
INCLUDING THE
? QUIZ-COMPENDS ?

CONTENTS.

	PAGE		PAGE
New Series of Manuals,	2,3,4,5	Obstetrics,	10
Anatomy,	6	Pathology, Histology,	11
Biology,	11	Pharmacy,	12
Chemistry,	6	Physiology,	11
Children's Diseases,	7	Practice of Medicine,	12
Dentistry,	8	Prescription Books,	12
Dictionaries,	8	? Quiz-Compends ?	14, 15
Eye Diseases,	8	Skin Diseases,	12
Electricity,	9	Surgery,	13
Gynæcology,	10	Therapeutics,	9
Hygiene,	9	Urine and Urinary Organs,	13
Materia Medica,	9	Venereal Diseases,	13
Medical Jurisprudence,	10		

PUBLISHED BY

P. BLAKISTON, SON & CO.,
Medical Booksellers, Importers and Publishers.

LARGE STOCK OF ALL STUDENTS' BOOKS, AT
THE LOWEST PRICES.

1012 Walnut Street, Philadelphia.

*** For sale by all Booksellers, or any book will be sent by mail, postpaid, upon receipt of price. Catalogues of books on all branches of Medicine, Dentistry, Pharmacy, etc., supplied upon application.

☞ Gould's New Medical Dictionary Just Ready. *See page 16.*

"An excellent Series of Manuals."—Archives of Gynæcology.

A NEW SERIES OF
STUDENTS' MANUALS

On the various Branches of Medicine and Surgery.

Can be used by Students of any College.

Price of each, Handsome Cloth, $3.00. Full Leather, $3.50.

The object of this series is to furnish good manuals for the medical student, that will strike the medium between the compend on one hand and the prolix text-book on the other—to contain all that is necessary for the student, without embarrassing him with a flood of theory and involved statements. They have been prepared by well-known men, who have had large experience as teachers and writers, and who are, therefore, well informed as to the needs of the student.

Their mechanical execution is of the best—good type and paper, handsomely illustrated whenever illustrations are of use, and strongly bound in uniform style.

Each book is sold separately at a remarkably low price, and the immediate success of several of the volumes shows that the series has met with popular favor.

No. 1. SURGERY. 236 Illustrations.

A Manual of the Practice of Surgery. By WM. J. WALSHAM, M.D., Asst. Surg. to, and Demonstrator of Surg. in, St. Bartholomew's Hospital, London, etc. 228 Illustrations.

Presents the introductory facts in Surgery in clear, precise language, and contains all the latest advances in Pathology, Antiseptics, etc.

"It aims to occupy a position midway between the pretentious manual and the cumbersome System of Surgery, and its general character may be summed up in one word—practical."—*The Medical Bulletin.*

"Walsham, besides being an excellent surgeon, is a teacher in its best sense, and having had very great experience in the preparation of candidates for examination, and their subsequent professional career, may be relied upon to have carried out his work successfully. Without following out in detail his arrangement, which is excellent, we can at once say that his book is an embodiment of modern ideas neatly strung together, with an amount of careful organization well suited to the candidate, and, indeed, to the practitioner."—*British Medical Journal.*

Price of each Book, Cloth, $3.00; Leather, $3.50.

No. 2. DISEASES OF WOMEN. 150 Illus.
NEW EDITION.

The Diseases of Women. Including Diseases of the Bladder and Urethra. By Dr. F. WINCKEL, Professor of Gynæcology and Director of the Royal University Clinic for Women, in Munich. Second Edition. Revised and Edited by Theophilus Parvin, M.D., Professor of Obstetrics and Diseases of Women and Children in Jefferson Medical College. 150 Engravings, most of which are original.

"The book will be a valuable one to physicians, and a safe and satisfactory one to put into the hands of students. It is issued in a neat and attractive form, and at a very reasonable price."—*Boston Medical and Surgical Journal.*

No. 3. OBSTETRICS. 227 Illustrations.

A Manual of Midwifery. By ALFRED LEWIS GALABIN, M.A., M.D., Obstetric Physician and Lecturer on Midwifery and the Diseases of Women at Guy's Hospital, London; Examiner in Midwifery to the Conjoint Examining Board of England, etc. With 227 Illus.

"This manual is one we can strongly recommend to all who desire to study the science as well as the practice of midwifery. Students at the present time not only are expected to know the principles of diagnosis, and the treatment of the various emergencies and complications that occur in the practice of midwifery, but find that the tendency is for examiners to ask more questions relating to the science of the subject than was the custom a few years ago. * * * The general standard of the manual is high; and wherever the science and practice of midwifery are well taught it will be regarded as one of the most important text-books on the subject."—*London Practitioner.*

No. 4. PHYSIOLOGY. Fourth Edition.
321 ILLUSTRATIONS AND A GLOSSARY

A Manual of Physiology. By GERALD F. YEO, M.D., F.R.C.S., Professor of Physiology in King's College, London. 321 Illustrations and a Glossary of Terms. Fourth American from second English Edition, revised and improved. 758 pages.

This volume was specially prepared to furnish students with a new text-book of Physiology, elementary so far as to avoid theories which have not borne the test of time and such details of methods as are unnecessary for students in our medical colleges.

"The brief examination I have given it was so favorable that I placed it in the list of text-books recommended in the circular of the University Medical College."—*Prof. Lewis A. Stimson*, M.D., *37 East 33d Street, New York.*

Price of each Book, Cloth, $3.00; Leather, $3.50.

No. 5. ORGANIC CHEMISTRY.

Or the Chemistry of the Carbon Compounds. By Prof. VICTOR VON RICHTER, University of Breslau. Authorized translation, from the Fourth German Edition. By EDGAR F. SMITH, M.A., PH.D.; Prof. of Chemistry in University of Pennsylvania; Member of the Chem. Socs. of Berlin and Paris.

"I must say that this standard treatise is here presented in a remarkably compendious shape."—*J. W. Holland*, M.D., *Professor of Chemistry, Jefferson Medical College, Philadelphia.*

"This work brings the whole matter, in simple, plain language, to the student in a clear, comprehensive manner. The whole method of the work is one that is more readily grasped than that of older and more famed text-books, and we look forward to the time when, to a great extent, this work will supersede others, on the score of its better adaptation to the wants of both teacher and student."—*Pharmaceutical Record.*

"Prof. von Richter's work has the merit of being singularly clear, well arranged, and for its bulk, comprehensive. Hence, it will, as we find it intimated in the preface, prove useful not merely as a text-book, but **as a manual of** reference."—*The Chemical News, London.*

No. 6. DISEASES OF CHILDREN.
SECOND EDITION.

A Manual. By J. F. GOODHART, M.D., Phys. to the Evelina Hospital for Children; Asst. Phys. to Guy's Hospital, London. Second American Edition. Edited and Rearranged by LOUIS STARR, M.D., Clinical Prof. of Dis. of Children in the Hospital of the Univ. of Pennsylvania, and Physician to the Children's Hospital, Phila. Containing many new Prescriptions, a list of over 50 Formulæ, conforming to the U. S. Pharmacopœia, and Directions for making Artificial Human Milk, for the Artificial Digestion of Milk, etc. Illus.

"The author has avoided the not uncommon error of writing a book on general medicine and labeling it 'Diseases of Children,' but has steadily kept in view the diseases which seemed to be incidental to childhood, or such points in disease as appear to be so peculiar to or pronounced in children as to justify insistence upon them. * * * A safe and reliable guide, and in many ways admirably adapted to the wants of the student and practitioner."—*American Journal of Medical Science.*

Price of each Book, Cloth, $3.00 ; Leather, $3.50.

THE NEW SERIES OF MANUALS. 5

No. 6. Goodhart and Starr:—Continued.

"Thoroughly individual, original and earnest, the work evidently of a close observer and an independent thinker, this book, though small, as a handbook or compendium is by no means made up of bare outlines or standard facts."—*The Therapeutic Gazette.*

"As it is said of some men, so it might be said of some books, that they are 'born to greatness.' This new volume has, we believe, a mission, particularly in the hands of the younger members of the profession. In these days of prolixity in medical literature, it is refreshing to meet with an author who knows both what to say and when he has said it. The work of Dr. Goodhart (admirably conformed, by Dr. Starr, to meet American requirements) is the nearest approach to clinical teaching without the actual presence of clinical material that we have yet seen."—*New York Medical Record.*

No. 7. PRACTICAL THERAPEUTICS.
FOURTH EDITION, WITH AN INDEX OF DISEASES.

Practical Therapeutics, considered with reference to Articles of the Materia Medica. Containing, also, an Index of Diseases, with a list of the Medicines applicable as Remedies. By EDWARD JOHN WARING, M.D., F.R.C.P. Fourth Edition. Rewritten and Revised by **DUDLEY** W. BUXTON, M.D., Asst. to the Prof. of Medicine at University College Hospital.

"We wish a copy could be put in the hands of every Student or Practitioner in the country. In our estimation, it is the best book of the kind ever written."—*N. Y. Medical Journal.*

No. 8. MEDICAL JURISPRUDENCE AND TOXICOLOGY.
NEW, REVISED AND ENLARGED EDITION.

By John J. Reese, M.D., Professor of Medical Jurisprudence and Toxicology in the University of Pennsylvania; President of the Medical Jurisprudence Society of Phila.; 2d Edition, Revised and Enlarged.

"This admirable text-book."—*Amer. Jour. of Med. Sciences.*
"We lay this volume aside, after a careful perusal of its pages, with the profound impression that it should be in the hands of every doctor and lawyer. It fully meets the wants of all students. . . . He has succeeded in admirably condensing into a handy volume all the essential points."—*Cincinnati Lancet and Clinic.*

Price of each Book, Cloth, $3,00; Leather, $3.50.

ANATOMY.

Macalister's Human Anatomy. 816 Illustrations. A new Text-book for Students and Practitioners, Systematic and Topographical, including the Embryology, Histology and Morphology of Man. With special reference to the requirements of Practical Surgery and Medicine. With 816 Illustrations, 400 of which are original. Octavo.   Cloth, 7.50 ; Leather, 8.50

Ballou's Veterinary Anatomy and Physiology. Illustrated. By Wm. R. Ballou, M.D., Professor of Equine Anatomy at New York College of Veterinary Surgeons. 29 graphic Illustrations. 12mo.   Cloth, 1.00 ; Interleaved for notes, 1.25

Holden's Anatomy. A manual of Dissection of the Human Body. Fifth Edition. Enlarged, with Marginal References and over 200 Illustrations. Octavo.   Cloth, 5.00 ; Leather, 6.00
    Bound in Oilcloth, for the Dissecting Room, $4.50.

"No student of Anatomy can take up this book without being pleased and instructed. Its Diagrams are original, striking and suggestive, giving more at a glance than pages of text description. * * * The text matches the illustrations in directness of practical application and clearness of detail."—*New York Medical Record.*

Holden's Human Osteology. Comprising a Description of the Bones, with Colored Delineations of the Attachments of the Muscles. The General and Microscopical Structure of Bone and its Development. With Lithographic Plates and Numerous Illustrations. Seventh Edition. 8vo.   Cloth, 6.00

Holden's Landmarks, Medical and Surgical. 4th ed. Clo., 1.25

Heath's Practical Anatomy. Sixth London Edition. 24 Colored Plates, and nearly 300 other Illustrations.   Cloth, 5.00

Potter's Compend of Anatomy. Fourth Edition. 117 Illustrations.   Cloth, 1.00 ; Interleaved for Notes, 1.25

CHEMISTRY.

Bartley's Medical Chemistry. Second Edition. A text-book prepared specially for Medical, Pharmaceutical and Dental Students. With 50 Illustrations, Plate of Absorption Spectra and Glossary of Chemical Terms. Revised and Enlarged. Cloth, 2.50

Trimble. Practical and Analytical Chemistry. A Course in Chemical Analysis, by Henry Trimble, Prof. of Analytical Chemistry in the Phila. College of Pharmacy. Illustrated. Third Edition. 8vo.   Cloth, 1.50

☞ *See pages 2 to 5 for list of Students' Manuals.*

STUDENTS' TEXT-BOOKS AND MANUALS. 7

Chemistry:—Continued.

Bloxam's Chemistry, Inorganic and Organic, with Experiments. Seventh Edition. Enlarged and Rewritten. 330 Illustrations.
Cloth, 4.50 ; Leather, 5.50

Richter's Inorganic Chemistry. A text-book for Students. Third American, from Fifth German Edition. Translated by Prof. Edgar F. Smith, PH.D. 89 Wood Engravings and Colored Plate of Spectra. Cloth, 2.00

Richter's Organic Chemistry, or Chemistry of the Carbon Compounds. Illustrated. Cloth, 3.00; Leather, 3.50

Symonds. Manual of Chemistry, for the special use of Medical Students. By BRANDRETH SYMONDS, A.M., M.D., Asst. Physician Roosevelt Hospital, Out-Patient Department; Attending Physician Northwestern Dispensary, New York. 12mo.
Cloth, 2.00 ; Interleaved for Notes, 2.40

Tidy. Modern Chemistry. 2d Ed. Cloth, 5.50

Leffmann's Compend of Chemistry. Inorganic and Organic. Including Urinary Analysis and the Sanitary Examination of Water. New Edition. Cloth, 1.00; Interleaved for Notes, 1.25

Muter. Practical and Analytical Chemistry. Second Edition, Revised and Illustrated. Cloth, 2.00

Holland. The Urine, Common Poisons, and Milk Analysis, Chemical and Microscopical. For Laboratory Use. 3d Edition, Enlarged. Illustrated. Cloth, 1.00

Van Nüys. Urine Analysis. Illus. Cloth, 2.00

Wolff's Applied Medical Chemistry. By Lawrence Wolff, M.D., Dem. of Chemistry in Jefferson Medical College. Clo., 1.00

CHILDREN.

Goodhart and Starr. The Diseases of Children. Second Edition. By J. F. Goodhart, M.D., Physician to the Evelina Hospital for Children; Assistant Physician to Guy's Hospital, London. Revised and Edited by Louis Starr, M.D., Clinical Professor of Diseases of Children in the Hospital of the University of Pennsylvania; Physician to the Children's Hospital, Philadelphia. Containing many Prescriptions and Formulæ, conforming to the U. S. Pharmacopœia, Directions for making Artificial Human Milk, for the Artificial Digestion of Milk, etc. Illustrated. Cloth, 3.00; Leather, 3.50

Hatfield. Diseases of Children. By M. P. Hatfield, M.D., Professor of Diseases of Children, Chicago Medical College. 12mo. Cloth, 1.00; Interleaved, 1.25

Day. On Children. A Practical and Systematic Treatise. Second Edition. 8vo. 752 pages. Cloth, 3.00; Leather, 4.00

☞ *See pages 14 and 15 for* **list** *of ? Quiz-Compends ?*

Children:—Continued.

Meigs and Pepper. The Diseases of Children. Seventh Edition. 8vo. Cloth, 5.00; Leather, 6.00

Starr. Diseases of the Digestive Organs in Infancy and Childhood. With chapters on the Investigation of Disease, and on the General Management of Children. By Louis Starr, M.D., Clinical Professor of Diseases of Children in the University of Pennsylvania; with a section on Feeding, including special Diet Lists, etc. Illus. Cloth, 2.50

DENTISTRY.

Fillebrown. Operative Dentistry. 330 Illus. Cloth, 2.50

Flagg's Plastics and Plastic Filling. 3d Ed. *Preparing.*

Gorgas. Dental Medicine. A Manual of Materia Medica and Therapeutics. Third Edition. Cloth, 3.50

Harris. Principles and Practice of Dentistry. Including Anatomy, Physiology, Pathology, Therapeutics, Dental Surgery and Mechanism. Twelfth Edition. Revised and enlarged by Professor Gorgas. 1028 Illustrations. Cloth, 7.00; Leather, 8.00

Richardson's Mechanical Dentistry. Fifth Edition. 569 Illustrations. 8vo. Cloth, 4.50; Leather, 5.50

Stocken's Dental Materia Medica. Third Edition. Cloth, 2.50

Taft's Operative Dentistry. Dental Students and Practitioners. Fourth Edition. 100 Illustrations. Cloth, 4.25; Leather, 5.00

Talbot. Irregularities of the Teeth, and their Treatment. Illustrated. 8vo. Cloth, 1.50

Tomes' Dental Anatomy. Third Ed. 191 Illus. Cloth, 4.00

Tomes' Dental Surgery. 3d Edition. Revised. 292 Illus. 772 Pages. Cloth, 5.00

DICTIONARIES.

Gould's New Medical Dictionary. Containing the Definition and Pronunciation of all words in Medicine, with many useful Tables etc. ½ Dark Leather, 3.25; ½ Mor., Thumb Index 4.25 *See last page.*

Cleaveland's Pocket Medical Lexicon. 31st Edition. Giving correct Pronunciation and Definition. Very small pocket size. Cloth, red edges .75; pocket-book style, 1.00

Longley's Pocket Dictionary. The Student's Medical Lexicon, giving Definition and Pronunciation of all Terms used in Medicine, with an Appendix giving Poisons and Their Antidotes, Abbreviations used in Prescriptions, Metric Scale of Doses, etc. 24mo. Cloth, 1.00; pocket-book style, 1.25

☞ *See pages 2 to 5 for list of Students' Manuals.*

EYE.

Arlt. Diseases of the Eye. Including those of the Conjunctiva, Cornea, Sclerotic, Iris and Ciliary Body. By Prof. Von Arlt. Translated by Dr. **Lyman Ware.** Illus. 8vo. Cloth, 2.50
Hartridge on Refraction. 4th Ed. Cloth, 2.00
Meyer. Diseases of the Eye. A complete Manual for Students and Physicians. 270 Illustrations and two Colored Plates. 8vo. Cloth, 4.50; Leather, 5.50
Fox and Gould. Compend of Diseases of the Eye and Refraction. 2d Ed. Enlarged. 71 Illus. 39 Formulæ.
Cloth, 1.00; Interleaved for Notes, 1.25

ELECTRICITY.

Mason's Compend of Medical and Surgical Electricity. With numerous Illustrations. 12mo. Cloth, 1.00

HYGIENE.

Parkes' (Ed. A.) Practical Hygiene. Seventh Edition, enlarged. Illustrated. 8vo. Cloth, 4.50
Parkes' (L. C.) Manual of Hygiene and Public Health. 12mo. Cloth, 2.50
Wilson's Handbook of Hygiene and Sanitary Science. Sixth Edition. Revised and Illustrated. Cloth, 2.75

MATERIA MEDICA AND THERAPEUTICS.

Potter's Compend of Materia Medica, Therapeutics and Prescription Writing. Fifth Edition, revised and improved.
Cloth, 1.00; Interleaved for Notes, 1.25
Biddle's Materia Medica. Eleventh Edition. By the late John B. Biddle, M.D., Professor of Materia Medica in Jefferson Medical College, Philadelphia. Revised, and rewritten, by Clement Biddle, M.D., Assist. Surgeon, U. S. N., assisted by Henry Morris, M.D. 8vo., illustrated. Cloth, 4.25; Leather, 5.00
Headland's Action of Medicines. 9th Ed. 8vo. Cloth, 3.00
Potter. Materia Medica, Pharmacy and Therapeutics. Including Action of Medicines, Special Therapeutics, Pharmacology, etc. Second Edition. Cloth, 4.00; Leather, 5.00
Starr, Walker and Powell. Synopsis of Physiological Action of Medicines, based upon Prof. H. C. Wood's "Materia Medica and Therapeutics." 3d Ed. Enlarged. Cloth, .75
Waring. Therapeutics. With an Index of Diseases and Remedies. 4th Edition. Revised. Cloth, 3.00; Leather, 3.50

☞ *See pages 14 and 15 for list of ? Quiz-Compends ?*

MEDICAL JURISPRUDENCE.

Reese. A Text-book of Medical Jurisprudence and Toxicology. By John J. Reese, M.D., Professor of Medical Jurisprudence and Toxicology in the Medical Department of the University of Pennsylvania; President of the Medical Jurisprudence Society of Philadelphia; Physician to St. Joseph's Hospital; Corresponding Member of The New York Medicolegal Society. 2d Edition. Cloth, 3.00; Leather, 3.50

Woodman and Tidy's Medical Jurisprudence and Toxicology. Chromo-Lithographic Plates and 116 Wood engravings.
Cloth, 7.50; Leather, 8.50

OBSTETRICS AND GYNÆCOLOGY.

Byford. Diseases of Women. The Practice of Medicine and Surgery, as applied to the Diseases and Accidents Incident to Women. By W. H. Byford, A.M., M.D., Professor of Gynæcology in Rush Medical College and of Obstetrics in the Woman's Medical College, etc., and Henry T. Byford, M.D., Surgeon to the Woman's Hospital of Chicago; Gynæcologist to St. Luke's Hospital, etc. Fourth Edition. Revised, Rewritten and Enlarged. With 306 Illustrations, over 100 of which are original. Octavo. 832 pages. Cloth, 5.00; Leather, 6.00

Cazeaux and Tarnier's Midwifery. With Appendix, by Mundé. The Theory and Practice of Obstetrics; including the Diseases of Pregnancy and Parturition, Obstetrical Operations, etc. By P. Cazeaux. Remodeled and rearranged, with revisions and additions, by S. Tarnier, M.D., Professor of Obstetrics and Diseases of Women and Children in the Faculty of Medicine of Paris. Eighth American, from the Eighth French and First Italian Edition. Edited by Robert J. Hess, M.D., Physician to the Northern Dispensary, Philadelphia, with an appendix by Paul F. Mundé, M.D., Professor of Gynæcology at the N. Y. Polyclinic. Illustrated by Chromo-Lithographs, Lithographs, and other Full-page Plates, seven of which are beautifully colored, and numerous Wood Engravings. *Students' Edition.* One Vol., 8vo. Cloth, 5.00; Leather, 6.00

Lewers' Diseases of Women. A Practical Text-Book. 139 Illustrations. Second Edition. Cloth, 2.50

Parvin's Winckel's Diseases of Women. Second Edition. Including a Section on Diseases of the Bladder and Urethra. 150 Illustrations. Revised. *See page 3.*
Cloth, 3.00; Leather, 3.50

Morris. Compend of Gynæcology. Illustrated. *In Press.*

Winckel's Obstetrics. A Text-book on Midwifery, including the Diseases of Childbed. By Dr. F. Winckel, Professor of Gynæcology, and Director of the Royal University Clinic for Women, in Munich. Authorized Translation, by J. Clifton Edgar, M.D., Lecturer on Obstetrics, University Medical College, New York, with nearly 200 handsome illustrations, the majority of which are original with this work. Octavo.
Cloth, 6.00; Leather, 7.00

Landis' Compend of Obstetrics. Illustrated. 4th edition, enlarged. Cloth, 1.00; Interleaved for Notes, 1.25

☞ *See pages 2 to 5 for list of New Manuals.*

STUDENTS' TEXT-BOOKS AND MANUALS. 11

Obstetrics and Gynæcology:—Continued.

Galabin's Midwifery. By A. Lewis Galabin, M.D., F.R.C.P. 227 Illustrations. *See page 3.* Cloth, 3.00; Leather, 3.50
Glisan's Modern Midwifery. 2d Edition. Cloth, 3.00
Rigby's Obstetric Memoranda. 4th Edition. Cloth, .50
Meadows' Manual of Midwifery. Including the Signs and Symptoms of Pregnancy, Obstetric Operations, Diseases of the Puerperal State, etc. 145 Illustrations. 494 pages. Cloth, 2.00
Swayne's Obstetric Aphorisms. For the use of Students commencing Midwifery Practice. 8th Ed. 12mo. Cloth, 1.25

PATHOLOGY. HISTOLOGY. BIOLOGY.

Bowlby. Surgical Pathology and Morbid Anatomy, for Students. 135 Illustrations. 12mo. Cloth, 2.00
Davis' Elementary Biology. Illustrated. Cloth, 4.00
Gilliam's Essentials of Pathology. A Handbook for Students. 47 Illustrations. 12mo. Cloth, 2.00

*** The object of this book is to unfold to the beginner the fundamentals of pathology in a plain, practical way, and by bringing them within easy comprehension to increase his interest in the study of the subject.

Gibbes' Practical Histology and Pathology. Third Edition. Enlarged. 12mo. Cloth, 1.75
Virchow's Post-Mortem Examinations. 2d Ed. Cloth, 1.00

PHYSIOLOGY.

Yeo's Physiology. Fourth Edition. The most Popular Students' Book. By Gerald F. Yeo, M.D., F.R.C.S., Professor of Physiology in King's College, London. Small Octavo. 758 pages. 321 carefully printed Illustrations. With a Full Glossary and Index. *See Page 3.* Cloth, 3.00; Leather, 3.50
Brubaker's Compend of Physiology. Illustrated. Fifth Edition. Cloth, 1.00; Interleaved for Notes, 1.25
Stirling. Practical Physiology, including Chemical and Experimental Physiology. 142 Illustrations. Cloth, 2.25
Kirke's Physiology. New 12th Ed. Thoroughly Revised and Enlarged. 502 Illustrations. Cloth, 4.00; Leather, 5.00
Landois' Human Physiology. Including Histology and Microscopical Anatomy, and with special reference to Practical Medicine. Third Edition. Translated and Edited by Prof. Stirling. 692 Illustrations. Cloth, 6.50; Leather, 7.50

"With this Text-book at his command, no student could fail in his examination."—*Lancet.*

Sanderson's Physiological Laboratory. Being Practical Exercises for the Student. 350 Illustrations. 8vo. Cloth, 5.00
Tyson's Cell Doctrine. Its History and Present State. Illustrated. Second Edition. Cloth, 2.00

☞ *See pages 14 and 15 for list of ? Quiz-Compends ?*

STUDENTS' TEXT-BOOKS AND MANUALS.

PRACTICE.

Taylor. Practice of Medicine. A Manual. By Frederick Taylor, M.D., Physician to, and Lecturer on Medicine at, Guy's Hospital, London; Physician to Evelina Hospital for Sick Children, and Examiner in Materia Medica and Pharmaceutical Chemistry, University of London. Cloth, 4.00

Roberts' Practice. New Revised Edition. A Handbook of the Theory and Practice of Medicine. By Frederick T. Roberts, M.D.; M.R.C.P., Professor of Clinical Medicine and Therapeutics in University College Hospital, London. **Seventh Edition.** Octavo. Cloth, 5.50; Sheep, 6.50

Hughes. Compend of the Practice of Medicine. 4th Edition. Two parts, each, Cloth, 1.00; Interleaved for Notes, 1.25

PART I.—Continued, Eruptive and Periodical Fevers, Diseases of the Stomach, Intestines, Peritoneum, Biliary Passages, Liver, Kidneys, etc., and General Diseases, etc.

PART II.—Diseases of the Respiratory System, Circulatory System and Nervous System; Diseases of the Blood, etc.

Physician's Edition. Fourth Edition. Including a Section on Skin Diseases. **With Index.** 1 vol. Full Morocco, Gilt, 2.50

Tanner's Index of Diseases, and Their Treatment. Cloth, 3.00

PRESCRIPTION BOOKS.

Wythe's Dose and Symptom Book. Containing the Doses and Uses of all the principal Articles of the Materia Medica, etc. Seventeenth Edition. Completely Revised and Rewritten. *Just Ready.* 32mo. Cloth, 1.00; Pocket-book style, 1.25

Pereira's Physician's Prescription Book. Containing Lists of Terms, Phrases, Contractions and Abbreviations used in Prescriptions Explanatory Notes, Grammatical Construction of Prescriptions, etc., etc. By Professor Jonathan Pereira, M.D. Sixteenth Edition. 32mo. Cloth, 1.00; Pocket-book style, 1.25

PHARMACY.

Stewart's Compend of Pharmacy. Based upon Remington's Text-Book of Pharmacy. Second Edition, Revised.
Cloth, 1.00; Interleaved for Notes, 1.25

SKIN DISEASES.

Anderson, (McCall) Skin Diseases. A complete Text-Book, with Colored Plates and numerous Wood Engravings. 8vo. *Just Ready.* Cloth, 4.50; Leather, 5.50

Van Harlingen on Skin Diseases. A Handbook of the Diseases of the Skin, their Diagnosis and Treatment (arranged alphabetically). By Arthur Van Harlingen, M.D., Clinical Lecturer on Dermatology, Jefferson Medical College; Prof. of Diseases of the Skin in the Philadelphia Polyclinic. 2d Edition. Enlarged. With colored and other plates and illustrations. 12mo. Cloth, 2.50

Bulkley. The Skin in Health and Disease. By L. Duncan Bulkley, Physician to the N. Y. Hospital. Illus. Cloth, .50

☞ *See pages 2 to 5 for list of New Manuals.*

SURGERY.

Caird and Cathcart. Surgical Handbook for the use of Practitioners and Students. By F. MITCHELL CAIRD, M.B., F.R.C.S., and C. WALKER CATHCART, M.B., F.R.C.S., Asst. Surgeons Royal Infirmary. With over 200 Illustrations. 400 pages. Pocket size. Leather covers, 2.50

Jacobson. Operations in Surgery. A Systematic Handbook for Physicians, Students and Hospital Surgeons. By W. H. A. Jacobson, B.A., Oxon. F.R.C.S. Eng.; Ass't Surgeon Guy's Hospital; Surgeon at Royal Hospital for Children and Women, etc. 199 Illustrations. 1006 pages. 8vo. Cloth. 5.00; Leather, 6.00

Heath's Minor Surgery, and Bandaging. Ninth Edition, 142 Illustrations. 60 Formulæ and Diet Lists. Cloth, 2.00

Horwitz's Compend of Surgery, including Minor Surgery, Amputations, Fractures, Dislocations, Surgical Diseases, and the Latest Antiseptic Rules, etc., with Differential Diagnosis and Treatment. By ORVILLE HORWITZ, B.S., M.D., Demonstrator of Surgery, Jefferson Medical College. 3d edition. Enlarged and Rearranged. 91 Illustrations and 77 Formulæ. 12mo.
  Cloth, 1.00; Interleaved for the addition of Notes, 1.25

Walsham. Manual of Practical Surgery. For Students and Physicians. By WM. J. WALSHAM, M.D., F.R.C.S., Asst. Surg. to, and Dem. of Practical Surg. in, St. Bartholomew's Hospital, Surgeon to Metropolitan Free Hospital, London. With 236 Engravings. *See Page 2.* Cloth, 3.00; Leather, 3.50

URINE, URINARY ORGANS, ETC.

Acton. The Reproductive Organs. In Childhood, Youth, Adult Life and Old Age. Seventh Edition. Cloth, 2.00

Beale. Urinary and Renal Diseases and Calculous Disorders. Hints on Diagnosis and Treatment. 12mo. Cloth, 1.75

Holland. The Urine, and Common Poisons and The Milk. Chemical and Microscopical, for Laboratory Use. Illustrated. Third Edition. 12mo. Interleaved. Cloth, 1.00

Ralfe. Kidney Diseases and Urinary Derangements. 42 Illustrations. 12mo. 572 pages. Cloth, 2.75

Legg. On the Urine. A Practical Guide. 6th Ed. Cloth, .75

Marshall and Smith. On the Urine. The Chemical Analysis of the Urine. By John Marshall, M.D., Chemical Laboratory, Univ. of Penna; and Prof. E. F. Smith, PH.D. Col. Plates. Cloth, 1.00

Thompson. Diseases of the Urinary Organs. Eighth London Edition. Illustrated. Cloth, 3.50

Tyson. On the Urine. A Practical Guide to the Examination of Urine. With Colored Plates and Wood Engravings. 6th Ed. Enlarged. 12mo. Cloth, 1.50

—— **Bright's Disease and Diabetes.** Illus. Cloth, 3.50

Van Nüys, Urine Analysis. Illus. Cloth, 2.00

VENEREAL DISEASES.

Hill and Cooper. Student's Manual of Venereal Diseases, with Formulæ. Fourth Edition. 12mo. Cloth, 1.00

Durkee. On Gonorrhœa and Syphilis. Illus. Cloth, 3.50

☞ *See pages 14 and 15 for list of ? Quiz-Compends ?*

NEW AND REVISED EDITIONS.

?QUIZ-COMPENDS?

The Best Compends for Students' Use in the Quiz Class, and when Preparing for Examinations.

Compiled in accordance with the latest teachings of prominent lecturers and the most popular Text-books.

They form a most complete, practical and exhaustive set of manuals, containing information nowhere else collected in such a condensed, practical shape. Thoroughly up to the times in every respect, containing many new prescriptions and formulæ, and over two hundred and fifty illustrations, many of which have been drawn and engraved specially for this series. The authors have had large experience as quiz-masters and attachés of colleges, with exceptional opportunities for noting the most recent advances and methods.

Cloth, each $1.00. Interleaved for Notes, $1.25.

No. 1. HUMAN ANATOMY, "Based upon Gray." Fourth Edition, including Visceral Anatomy, formerly published separately. Over 100 Illustrations. By SAMUEL O. L. POTTER, M.A., M.D., late A. A. Surgeon U. S. Army. Professor of Practice, Cooper Medical College, San Francisco.

Nos. 2 and 3. PRACTICE OF MEDICINE. Fourth Edition. By DANIEL E. HUGHES, M.D., Demonstrator of Clinical Medicine in Jefferson Medical College, Philadelphia. In two parts.

PART I.—Continued, Eruptive and Periodical Fevers, Diseases of the Stomach, Intestines, Peritoneum, Biliary Passages, Liver, Kidneys, etc. (including Tests for Urine), General Diseases, etc.

PART II.—Diseases of the Respiratory System (including Physical Diagnosis), Circulatory System and Nervous System; Diseases of the Blood, etc.

** These little books can be regarded as a full set of notes upon the Practice of Medicine, containing the Synonyms, Definitions, Causes, Symptoms, Prognosis, Diagnosis, Treatment, etc., of each disease, and including a number of prescriptions hitherto unpublished.

No. 4. PHYSIOLOGY, including Embryology. Fifth Edition. By ALBERT P. BRUBAKER, M.D., Prof. of Physiology, Penn'a College of Dental Surgery; Demonstrator of Physiology in Jefferson Medical College, Philadelphia. Revised, Enlarged and Illustrated.

No. 5. OBSTETRICS. Illustrated. Fourth Edition. By HENRY G. LANDIS, M.D., Prof. of Obstetrics and Diseases of Women, in Starling Medical College, Columbus, O. Revised Edition. New Illustrations.

BLAKISTON'S ? QUIZ-COMPENDS ?
Continued.

Bound in Cloth, $1.00.   Interleaved, for Notes, $1.25

No. 6. MATERIA MEDICA, THERAPEUTICS AND PRESCRIPTION WRITING. Fifth Revised Edition With especial Reference to the Physiological Action of Drugs, and a complete article on Prescription Writing. Based on the Last Revision of the U. S. Pharmacopœia, and including many unofficinal remedies. By SAMUEL O. L. POTTER, M.A., M.D., late A. A. Surg. U. S. Army; Prof. of Practice, Cooper Medical College, San Francisco. Improved and Enlarged, with Index.

No. 7. GYNÆCOLOGY. A Compend of Diseases of Women. By HENRY MORRIS, M.D., Demonstrator of Obstetrics, Jefferson Medical College, Philadelphia.

No. 8. DISEASES OF THE EYE AND REFRACTION, including Treatment and Surgery. By L. WEBSTER FOX, M.D., Chief Clinical Assistant Ophthalmological Dept., Jefferson Medical College, etc., and GEO. M. GOULD, M.D. 71 Illustrations, 39 Formulæ. Second Enlarged and Improved Edition. Index.

No. 9. SURGERY. Illustrated. Third Edition. Including Fractures, Wounds, Dislocations, Sprains, Amputations and other operations; Inflammation, Suppuration, Ulcers, Syphilis, Tumors, Shock, etc. Diseases of the Spine, Ear, Bladder, Testicles, Anus, and other Surgical Diseases. By ORVILLE HORWITZ, A.M., M.D., Demonstrator of Surgery, Jefferson Medical College. Revised and Enlarged. 77 Formulæ and 91 Illustrations.

No. 10. CHEMISTRY. Inorganic and Organic. For Medical and Dental Students. Including Urinary Analysis and Medical Chemistry. By HENRY LEFFMANN, M.D., Prof. of Chemistry in Penn'a College of Dental Surgery, Phila. Third Edition, Revised and Rewritten, with Index.

No. 11. PHARMACY. Based upon "Remington's Text-book of Pharmacy." By F. E. STEWART, M.D., PH.G., Quiz-Master at Philadelphia College of Pharmacy. Second Edition, Revised.

No. 12. VETERINARY ANATOMY AND PHYSIOLOGY. 29 Illustrations. By WM. R. BALLOU, M.D., Prof. of Equine Anatomy at N. Y. College of Veterinary Surgeons.

No. 13. DISEASES OF CHILDREN. By DR. MARCUS P. HATFIELD, Prof. of Diseases of Children, Chicago Medical College.

Bound in Cloth, $1.   Interleaved, for the Addition of Notes, $1.25.

☞ *These books* **are constantly revised to keep up with the latest teachings** *and discoveries, so that they contain all the new methods and principles.* **No series of books are so complete in detail, concise in language, or so well printed and bound. Each** *one* **forms a complete set of notes upon the subject under consideration.**

Descriptive Circular Free.

NOW READY.

A NEW MEDICAL DICTIONARY.

BY GEORGE M. GOULD,

Ophthalmic Surgeon, Philadelphia Hospital, etc.

AN ENTIRELY NEW BOOK.

BASED ON RECENT MEDICAL LITERATURE.

Small Octavo. 520 Pages. Handsomely Printed.

Bound in Half Dark Leather, $3.25.

Half Morocco, Thumb Index, $4.25.

SEND FOR SPECIAL CIRCULAR.

JUST PUBLISHED.

A NEW
MEDICAL DICTIONARY,

BY

GEORGE M. GOULD, A.B., M.D.,

OPHTHALMIC SURGEON TO THE PHILADELPHIA HOSPITAL, CLINICAL CHIEF OPHTHALMOLOGICAL DEPT. GERMAN HOSPITAL, PHILADELPHIA.

A compact, concise Vocabulary, including **all the Words and Phrases used in medicine**, with their proper Pronunciation and Definitions,

BASED ON RECENT MEDICAL LITERATURE.

It is **not a** mere compilation from other dictionaries. The definitions have been made by the aid of the most recent standard text-books in the various branches of medicine, and it will therefore meet the wants of **every** physician and student. It includes

SEVERAL THOUSAND WORDS NOT CONTAINED IN ANY SIMILAR WORK.

It is printed on handsome paper, made especially for the purpose; **from a new type** selected on account of its clear, distinct **face, and** is bound so that it will lie **open** at any page.

Small Octavo, 520 Pages, Half-Dark Leather, $3.25. With Thumb Index, Half Morocco, Marbled Edges, $4.25.

It may be obtained through Booksellers, Wholesale Druggists and Dental Depots everywhere.

[OVER]

FROM PROF. J. M. DACOSTA: "I find it an excellent work, doing credit to the learning and discrimination of the author."

GOULD'S NEW MEDICAL DICTIONARY.

There has been no dictionary accessible to the physician and student that has kept pace with the coinage of new words and terms during the past ten years. The growth of specialism in itself has increased the vocabulary by some thousands of words; and yet the busy practitioner or student has been offered no compact, thorough dictionary to which he could turn for a definition absolutely necessary to the proper understanding of the article he might be reading.

This expressed want has led to the preparation of this work. The aim has been to prepare a handbook of sufficient scope to include everything of use to the general practitioner and student, and at the same time to be a compact, handy volume, giving the exact information desired at a quick reference. The wants of the specialist have also been taken into consideration, and the seeker after more extended knowledge will find much precise information relating to his special branch, to the etymology and meaning of words, etc.

IT CONTAINS TABLES

1. Of the **ABBREVIATIONS** used in Medicine, Prefixes and Suffixes of Medical Words, etc.
2. Of the ARTERIES, with the Name, Origin, Distribution and Branches of each.
3. Of the BACILLI, giving the Name, Habitat, Characteristics of the Cultures (upon slides, gelatin, gelose, potato and bouillon). Description of the Cellules, the Influence of Oxygen and Heat, the Physiological Action, and Sundry Observations.
4. Of GANGLIA, with the Name, Location, Roots and Distribution of each.
5. Of LEUCOMAINES, giving the Name, Formula, Discoverer, Source and Physiological Action.
6. Of MICROCOCCI, giving the same information as in the case of the Bacilli.
7. Of **MUSCLES**, with the Name, Origin, Insertion, Innervation **and** Function.
8. Of NERVES, with the Name, Function, Origin, Distribution and Branches.
9. Of PLEXUSES, with the Name, Location, Derivation and Distribution.
10. Of PTOMAINES, with the Name, **Formula**, Discoverer, Source and Physiological Action.
11. Of COMPARISON OF THERMOMETERS; of all the most used WEIGHTS AND MEASURES of the world; of the MINERAL SPRINGS OF THE U. S., VITAL STATISTICS, etc., etc.

Some of the material thus classified is not obtainable by English readers in any other work.

[OVER]

"The compact size of this Dictionary, its clear type, and its accuracy are unfailing pointers to its coming popularity."
—*John B. Hamilton, Surgeon-General U. S. Marine Hospital Service.*

www.ingramcontent.com/pod-product-compliance
Lightning Source LLC
Chambersburg PA
CBHW022113160426
43197CB00009B/1009